Active Management of Labour

The Dublin Experience

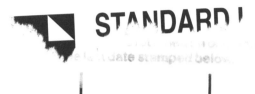

Active Management of Labour

The Dublin Experience

Third edition

Kieran O'Driscoll
Declan Meagher

with

Peter Boylan

National Maternity Hospital
& University College Dublin

Mosby

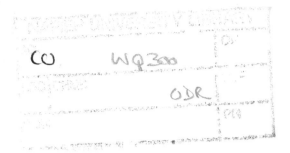

Copyright © Mosby Year book Europe Limited, 1993
Published by Mosby Year book Europe Limited, 1993
Printed and bound in Great Britain by BPCC Hazells Ltd,
Aylesbury, England

ISBN 0 7234 1910 8

A CIP catalogue record for this book is available from the British
Library.

For full details of all Mosby–Year Book Europe Limited titles please
write to Mosby–Year Book Europe Limited, Brook House, 2–16
Torrington Place, London WC1E 7LT, England.

DEDICATED TO THE NURSING STAFF
IN THE DELIVERY UNIT OF THE
NATIONAL MATERNITY HOSPITAL IN
RECOGNITION OF THEIR UNFAILING
COOPERATION AT ALL TIMES

Contents

Preface

The Third Edition of this book continues to be firmly based on personal experience of everyday clinical practice in a large obstetric unit with extensive teaching commitments. The original motivation, which was to enhance the experience of childbirth for mothers with none of the textbook abnormalities, remains substantially unchanged. The format too stays the same. Because the seemingly inexorable rise in caesarean birth rates has come to represent a public health issue of major proportions in many countries, the comparatively low surgical delivery rate maintained in this institution over the years has attracted considerable attention at international level. It seems fitting to emphasise, therefore, that these low surgical delivery rates were not pursued as an end in themselves, but emerged as a reflection of labour management. It is a pleasure to acknowledge our indebtedness to Dr Dermot MacDonald (Master 1977–1983) and Dr Niall O'Brien (Consultant Paediatrician) and to Dr Adrian Grant of the National Perinatal Epidemiology Unit at Oxford, for permission to abstract from what has become generally known as the Dublin Trial of the comparative value of electronic fetal heart monitors, expressed in terms of immediate survival and in terms of cerebral palsy after 4 years of age. This classical study is freely drawn upon in chapters 23 and 28; reference to the complete texts, which are cited in the List of Publications, is strongly recommended. The statistical data for the hospital are updated to 1990; we are grateful to Dr John Stronge (Master 1984–1990) for permission to include the most recent figures.

Kieran O'Driscoll   *Declan Meagher*

Peter Boylan
Master
1991–

Preface to the First Edition

The authors are indebted to very many persons, too numerous to mention, for advice over the years. First, it must be said that a project of this nature could not even have been contemplated without the wholehearted cooperation of the Nursing Sisters in the delivery unit, whose high standards of professional achievement were matched by a flexible attitude to new ideas to a degree that made everything possible. Likewise, our junior medical colleagues, who occupied the position of Assistant Master and whose names have appeared as co-authors of several publications in the medical press: they shared the responsibility for the welfare of every woman and child delivered and made many contributions to the underlying philosophy. And our medical colleagues farther afield, of whom a few only are mentioned here by name, because they made specific recommendations which we have incorporated as standard practice in the management of labour: Dr E.A. Friedman for the graphic representation of cervical dilatation, Dr R.H. Philpott for the introduction of an action-line, and Dr C.H. Hendricks for the suggestions that the duration of labour be measured from the time of admission to a delivery unit. We also wish to acknowledge our debt to the staff of the Physiotherapy Department and to the staff of the Medical Records Department for valuable assistance through the years. Finally, we are grateful to Dr Dermot MacDonald, presently Master of the National Maternity Hospital, for his encouragement in this undertaking.

Kieran O'Driscoll
Master
1963–1969

Declan Meagher
Master
1970–1976

Introduction

The purpose of this manual is to present the principles, the practice and the results of active management of labour as it has evolved at the National Maternity Hospital Dublin over a period in excess of 25 years. The contents represent the fruits of the personal experience of the authors who as Masters, each for a duration of seven years, were directly responsible for 100,000 births and who for the intervening years were closely involved with an additional 100,000 births – a total of some 200,000 births overall. The text encompasses a comprehensive approach to the conduct of labour as put into effect several times every day in one of the largest obstetric units in the British Isles. This is not an academic exercise nor a review of literature.

The contents are addressed primarily to obstetricians and midwives, as the people most closely involved with the provision of high standards of care in labour, but are hardly less relevant to anaesthetists, childbirth educators, physiotherapists and, indeed, to others who strive towards this common end. Also, as no expert knowledge is needed to comprehend the universal significance of the principles enunciated, the text is eminently suitable for medical students and student midwives in contact with the birth process for the first time. Although the principles of active management of labour remain valid in all circumstances, the practice should be considered only in the context of a suitable hospital environment, never in the home.

Background

Although childbirth has long ceased to present a serious physical challenge to healthy women in western society, the emotional impact of labour remains a matter of common concern. In orthodox medical circles recognition has come slowly that labour, especially first labour, may be the most disturbing emotional event in the lifetime of one-half of humankind. Failure to place nearly enough emphasis on this aspect of the subject is often attributed to the fact that obstetricians are mostly men, although midwives, as women, have shown no greater insight. Rather, the correct explanation seems to us to be that for far too long there has been a tacit acceptance of the conservative, or passive, attitude to labour where nothing could be done to resolve an admittedly unpleasant situation without the introduction of serious extraneous hazards with possible adverse effects on both mother and child. According to this viewpoint, which still gains wide credence, there is no safe alternative to the well-tried doctrine of watchful expectancy – but only to a point: the point of full dilatation. The doctrine of watchful expectancy covers the tedious hours of the first stage of labour until the cervix reaches full dilatation. At this point the outlook tends to change dramatically, so that almost any procedure aimed at vaginal delivery becomes acceptable.

This sudden change, from an extremely conservative approach to the first stage, to an equally radical approach to the second stage, epitomises passive management of labour, which the authors have long since abandoned. As might be expected from the foregoing account, passive management of labour is marked also by the emphasis placed on drugs to relieve pain during the extended first stage, and on the acquisition of manual skills to procure vaginal delivery once the cervix ceases to present an obstacle.

As the problem of maternal mortality has receded further into history, medical attention has been transferred to the child. Perinatal mortality and, to an increasing degree, perinatal morbidity have become the touchstones of modern obstetrics. One result of this change is that labour, nowadays, is made even more arduous for mothers by the introduction of invasive procedures undertaken in the name of the child, often with scant evidence about their real value. Somehow the idea seems to have gained ground that a conflict of interest necessarily exists between mother and child during labour and that mothers can be subjected to almost any form of indignity or any degree of discomfort provided this is well-intentioned and undertaken on behalf of the child. We certainly do not subscribe to this proposition: on the contrary, our experience suggests that what is good for mothers is good for babies too, especially where short duration of labour and delivery without trauma are concerned. A main aim of this manual is to redress the rapidly growing imbalance in the birth process to favour the mother, without detriment to her child.

As long ago as 1963 a concerted effort was begun to improve the quality of care extended to all women in labour in this hospital. It so happens that this hospital is in an exceptionally favourable position to embark on such a project, for two main reasons: first, in numerical terms, it is one of the largest maternity units in the British Isles and, second, one obstetrician is ultimately responsible for the welfare of all mothers and babies. These inherent advantages afford a unique opportunity to establish a uniform pattern of care in a large number of cases. Two additional features are worthy of note: dead babies are almost invariably submitted to expert post-mortem examination and live babies with evidence of cerebral dysfunction are retained on permanent record. Finally, there is an efficient system of medical records which is reflected in the timely publication of an Annual Clinical Report with extensive international circulation. A continuous internal medical audit system ensures that every important aspect of obstetric practice is kept under constant review, so that labour is not considered as a subject in isolation from all other aspects of childbirth, such as caesarean section, the incidence of which has shown little change over these years.

Meanwhile, a growing tendency to resolve the problems of the first stage of labour by surgical intervention has resulted in an alarming increase in the number of caesarean sections performed in most other centres. Caesarean section rates are currently the most realistic objective measure of the standard of obstetric care afforded to mothers, replacing maternal mortality rates, which are outmoded for this purpose in developed countries. By this criterion the overall standard of care afforded to mothers has declined markedly in recent times. Perinatal mortality rates must continue to serve the same purpose in infants until such time as morbidity rates are sufficiently clearly defined.

Procedure

Before any worthwhile improvement in the conduct of labour could even be contemplated, it was evident that the person ultimately responsible must return to the delivery unit to assume direct responsibility for the welfare of all mothers, not just in theory but also in practice. Whereas previously the consultant obstetrician had been invoked only in a small number of abnormal cases of eclampsia, breech presentation or diabetes mellitus, who happened to be in labour, he must now become involved directly with the much larger number of perfectly normal women who had hitherto been overlooked at consultant level because they suffered from neither obstetrical complication nor organic disease. Furthermore, it is clear that this commitment must begin at admission and continue until delivery. The consultant, rather than remaining off-stage awaiting the occasional summons to perform an emergency operation in a belated attempt to retrieve a situation which could have been anticipated at a much earlier stage, must seek to prevent such emergencies arising in women who were normal when first admitted to hospital in labour. Ironically, it is in completely normal women that most of the problems of labour arise.

The position of the Sister, or senior midwife in charge of the delivery unit, was seen as a matter of no less importance. Although closely involved at all stages of labour hitherto, she had remained largely powerless to influence the course of events. Apart from the administration of analgesic drugs, possibly, she lacked clear guidance on how to proceed when storm clouds began to gather. Yet in spite of this anomaly she was constantly exposed to the possibility of unfair criticism from either side. These genuine grievances had contributed to a generally low state of morale among nursing staff, and they remain one of the root causes of relatively poor standards of overall patient care in many delivery units. One of the most important issues raised in this publication is an urgent need to define the professional relationships which should exist between doctors and midwives at different levels of experience. Only when this issue is resolved in a mutually satisfactory manner will it be possible to develop the genuine team spirit which is an essential feature of an efficient service. Adoption of good resolutions to improve the quality of care offered to all women in labour, is worthless without the unqualified cooperation of nursing staff because, in the final analysis, it is nursing staff who must convert resolutions into practice.

From the outset, the delivery unit in this hospital was designated an intensive care area, wherein every woman and unborn child must be reviewed by a competent medical officer, in the company of the midwife in charge, at regular intervals, especially late at night and early in the morning. The official record of each individual delivered during the previous 24 hours was made the object of special scrutiny by the authors and a current account of the main events was maintained on a daily basis. In this way the consultant obstetrician became actively involved in the conduct of labour on a regular basis as never before. Hence, the origin of the term active management of labour. The word 'active', in this context, refers to the nature of the involvement of the consultant obstetrician; it certainly is not intended to convey to the reader that he intervenes more often. Indeed, precisely the opposite is the case, as the unusually low figures for all forms of operative intervention clearly illustrate. Active participation in the day to day functions of the delivery unit of the person ultimately responsible, opened entirely new prospects on labour management; these have led to a fundamental reappraisal of almost all the conventional wisdoms. Many proved false. Although not apparently based on any factual evidence, these had been relayed from teacher to student and textbook to textbook without any serious attempt at verification, until they had come to represent possibly the main impediment to progress in the field.

As a result of this extensive personal and carefully documented experience, management of labour is now based squarely on the simple proposition that efficient uterine action is the key to normality. A strictly pragmatic approach has shown beyond doubt that efficient uterine action can be provided with a very high degree of safety, subject to a small number of rules which are precisely stated. As a consequence of these new-found certainties, a dynamic approach to the birth process, based on efficient uterine action, has replaced the old static approach based largely on pelvic architecture. What may aptly be described as the domino effect of efficient uterine action has left no aspect of labour untouched and, in particular, has brought about a situation in which every expectant mother who attends this hospital for antenatal care is given two firm assurances, to the effect that labour will not last longer than 12 hours and that she will never be left without a personal nurse by her side at all times. These two virtual guarantees have changed the face of women's expectations of labour. Taken together they come close to the kernel of the problem of labour management, while in practice they remain entirely dependent on each other.

Presentation

This manual is divided into three sections.

Section I

The main text consists of a description of the aspects of labour which the authors consider to be of such fundamental importance that each must be examined in considerable detail before any genuine progress can be made. These items are named in the Contents and special notice should be paid to the list of chapter headings, because these are topics not often discussed in standard textbooks. Not one of these items can be safely omitted because, like the various pieces of a jigsaw puzzle, they fit snugly together to form a composite picture of which no one fragment can stand alone. The language used is both simple and direct. Technical and Latinate terms are purposely avoided because they frequently serve as a cloak to obscure lack of true meaning.

In the opening chapters particular attention is directed to the absolute need to distinguish clearly between first and all subsequent births, between induction of labour and acceleration of labour that has already started, and to the fact that obstetrical abnormalities – specifically malpresentations, malformation and twins – must always be excluded before consideration can be given to management of labour as a distinct entity. Hence this manual is concerned solely with the prototypal woman in labour: the primigravida with vertex presentation and single fetus. In subsequent chapters the basic parameters of labour are carefully defined and the rules which govern the use of oxytocin to accelerate progress when labour is slow are stated in quite explicit terms.

In later chapters the causes of abnormal labour are examined, and in the course of this examination the conventional deference shown to cephalopelvic disproportion, which had so dominated attitudes towards labour in former times, is totally rejected. Several chapters are devoted to consideration of the age-old problem of maternal stress, and here the emphasis is on communication as a vital ingredient of good labour management. Drugs are said to play but a minor, and largely unsatisfactory, role.

The closing chapters are concerned with the organisation of a busy delivery unit where medical efficiency and human compassion can exist side by side. Organisation is regarded as a matter of fundamental importance on which all else must ultimately depend. Indeed, poor organisation is identified as the rock on which good intentions, in the medical sphere, most often founder.

A chapter on induction of labour is included, in the somewhat vain hope that it may serve to dispel at least some of the obfuscation which bedevils this topic; another chapter deals with the relationship between effacement and dilatation of cervix, since these expressions are in constant use but seldom accurately defined. Then there is the matter of caesarean section rates which seem sure to develop into one of the most contentious medical issues of our time. Finally, the tragedy of cerebral palsy, which for various reasons has come to cast a threatening shadow over the whole question of labour management, is examined in the context of the practice set down in these pages.

A few terms may benefit from definition because of different interpretation in other centres: primigravida or nullipara refers to a woman who has not previously given birth to a viable infant; nurse and midwife are synonymous as both are state registered nurses and either trained or student midwives; a senior registrar requires a specialist qualification in obstetrics and gynaecology, whereas a resident medical officer is in the process of training.

Section II

The second section consists of a series of visual case records, each selected to illustrate one important aspect of labour, with a brief explanatory
note on the facing page. These visual records, or partographs, illustrate
better than words ever can, the problems that arise in the course of
everyday practice. Together they constitute an identikit with which it is
possible to construct an endless variety of profiles of labour, to meet
almost any clinical circumstance. The authors regard this as the most
instructive section of the book, because by concentrating the mind it
involves the reader directly in the study of labour as a concrete, rather
than an abstract, pursuit.

The design and content of these visual records are matters which have
an immediate impact on the conduct of labour. The model used in this
hospital is worthy of close attention because it is the final product of several years of gradual development in the light of personal experience
gained on the floor of a busy delivery unit. Simplicity is the keynote:
every detail not immediately relevant to the main issue is rigorously
excluded. The graph which portrays progress dominates the picture and
no provision is made for labour to last longer than 12 hours. Two colours
are used to separate primigravidae from multigravidae. This is a basic
requirement. The point is emphasised again and again in the course of
the text. A loose leaf arrangement facilitates retention of all visual
records of labour in two clip-in folders, one for primigravidae and one
for multigravidae. These are retained in the delivery unit where they are
available for inspection and discussion. This simple device allows a continuous audit of all the relevant items, which in turn provides a very
effective method of central control of the entire service.

The educational potential of these case records is limitless. They have
made a unique contribution to the general understanding of the birth
process in this hospital and have proved an invaluable aid in the education of both doctors and nurses, and indeed mothers too; mothers perhaps most of all, because they are used as the focus of antenatal preparation for labour. In addition, they continue to provide fertile ground for
clinical research and for graduate seminars which can be conducted like
exercises in map reading, where abstract names become real places as
soon as they are located in relation to the surrounding terrain. A serious
student can quickly compile a personal series of case records to illustrate
the whole gamut of labour experience and in the process construct a
storehouse of practical information. Success in this direction is determined by the ability of visual records to speak for themselves and thus
reflect a live and durable portrait of one woman and her child in labour.

Section III

The third section consists of a summary of the clinical material which
passed through the National Maternity Hospital during the years when
active management of labour became standard practice. This information
provides the factual background to the text. As events in labour seldom

happen in isolation, action taken in one direction is likely to have repercussions in another. Thus, to restrict the duration of labour to 12 hours would serve no useful purpose were this to be achieved at the expense of a significant increase in the incidence of caesarean section in the case of the mother, and mortality or morbidity in the case of the child. The facts will enable readers to see for themselves that statements made in the text are not based on purely theoretical considerations. They also enable comparisons to be made with results from other centres. Best of all, the figures demonstrate the balance that has been struck between one outcome of labour and another. Information of this scope is too often missing from publications which are confined to one narrow aspect of labour: epidural anaesthesia is one of many such examples. This form of selective reporting can conceal a significant underlying distortion in the overall picture.

The authors see no good reason why the results presented here should not be reproduced in other centres. This does not mean that comparable results can be achieved overnight; many delivery units are so completely disorganised that there is no possibility of their providing an efficient service as they presently function. Dublin women are not different, only better educated, in the sense that they comprehend the simple logic of the procedure described in these pages because it has been lucidly explained to them beforehand. This has nothing whatever to do with regimentation: it is a matter of plain common sense.

Publications on the subject of labour which emanated from the National Maternity Hospital during the same period are listed on page 211. These correspond broadly with the chapter headings.

In conclusion, the authors recommend strongly that the pages of this manual be read through consecutively, from beginning to end.

Section I

1: Primigravidae v Multigravidae

There are fundamental differences between a first and all subsequent births. These differences are so great that they warrant the statement that primigravidae and multigravidae behave as different biological species. The precise nature of the differences between primigravidae and multigravidae must be appreciated before management of labour can be established on any semblance of a rational basis.[1]

To ensure that the fundamental differences between a first and a subsequent birth are kept constantly in mind in this hospital, the same labour record is printed on two colours: yellow for primigravidae and blue for multigravidae. The result is that the first item of information which confronts even the most casual observer is that a woman in labour has, or has not, had a previous birth. This remarkably simple device has had a major impact on labour management. (See *Graphs 1* and *28*.)

Unique experience

Modern management of labour, as it relates to welfare of mothers, is concerned primarily with emotional rather than with physical stress. Labour represents a significant physical challenge to very few women in contemporary practice, and these individuals are generally identified beforehand because they suffer from systemic diseases. The birth of a first child, however, is almost surely the most profound emotional experience, for good or ill, in an average lifetime. The first experience is of paramount importance because it determines the attitude to all subsequent births.

A woman who has a happy first experience is unlikely to suffer much apprehension about a later birth, whereas a woman who has had an unhappy first experience is likely to be terrified at the prospect of a repeat performance. These fears can have grave consequences outside the narrow confines of obstetrics; they can haunt a woman for the rest of her life, and affect her attitude to her husband and also possibly to her child. Typically, the residual effect of an unhappy first experience is revealed in a second pregnancy by an urgent request for epidural anaesthesia, as an opening gambit at the initial antenatal visit, in the firm expectation that the previous ordeal is likely to be repeated. Prompt accession to this request reinforces the fear, for which there is absolutely no foundation in clinical practice. A first labour is unique; the sequence of events which takes place on that occasion has no relevance to later births. The lesson is simple: provide a high standard of care and attention first time round and a woman will require little assistance on the next occasion. Conversely, the damage inflicted by a low standard of care and attention first time round is usually irreversible.

Prolonged labour

The most distinctive feature of first labour is duration. A first labour is longer, because inefficient uterine action is common and because the genital tract has not been stretched before. This applies equally to the cervix in the first stage and to the vagina in the second stage. Slow progress in a primigravida should always be regarded as an expression of inefficient uterine action; the possibility of cephalopelvic disproportion should not even be entertained until efficient uterine action has been assured.

The duration of subsequent labour is comparatively short, partly because inefficient uterine action is a rare occurrence in multigravidae, and partly because the genital tract has been stretched on a previous occasion. Slow progress in labour in a parous woman should never be assumed to be an expression of inefficient uterine action, but rather an expression of obstruction caused by a fetal complication, such as malpresentation or malformation. This obstruction can easily lead to rupture of uterus in a parous woman, especially if oxytocin is used to expedite delivery.

Cephalopelvic disproportion

Another distinctive feature of first labour is cephalopelvic disproportion. This possibility arises simply because the functional capacity of the pelvis is not yet known. Hence, the term cephalopelvic disproportion should be restricted to primigravidae, to avoid confusion with obstructed labour in multigravidae in whom the functional capacity of the pelvis is already proven. Obstructed labour, in a parous woman, is a different clinical entity altogether and it is fraught with far more sinister consequences for both mother and child. Cephalopelvic disproportion is linked, erroneously, in the collective subconscious of obstetricians, with fear of serious injury to mother and child. This mistaken association of ideas has greatly impeded improvements in the management of labour for many years.

Rupture of uterus

Another distinctive feature of first labour is immunity to rupture. Rupture of uterus is such an exceptional event in primigravidae that for practical purposes it can be assumed not to occur. The sole exception is manipulation. Serious injury to a primigravida, of which rupture of uterus is the ultimate example, is inflicted usually with instruments. This is one of the most important clinical observations in the entire field of obstetrics. In particular, this observation has led us to a complete reappraisal of the hitherto general assumption that oxytocin may cause rupture of uterus in the presence of undetected cephalopelvic disproportion. There is now ample evidence that this assumption, which has dominated the conduct of labour for so long, has no foundation in practice. There can be no doubt whatever that the mistake arose from failure to draw a sufficiently clear distinction between primigravidae and multigravidae in labour. Indeed, the fear that oxytocin may cause rupture of uterus is only too well founded in multigravidae: whereas primigravidae are rupture proof, multigravidae are rupture prone. The inherent tendency of the multigravid uterus to rupture is a factor which must be taken into account whenever the potential risks of epidural anaesthesia are under consideration.

Traumatic intracranial haemorrhage

Yet another distinctive feature of first labour is the likelihood of serious injury to the child. Rupture of tentorium cerebelli, with consequent subdural haemorrhage, is the extreme example. This lesion corresponds with rupture of uterus in the mother. Rupture of tentorium occurs during the second stage of labour and, in cephalic presentation, it is almost invariably associated with instrumental delivery. Consequently, serious injury to the child occurs much more often in primigravidae, not because of cephalopelvic disproportion but because of the comparatively high incidence of forceps delivery. The influence of epidural anaesthesia is relevant in this context.

Extensive experience with oxytocin to ensure efficient uterine action in primigravidae has shown that the risk of serious injury to both mother and child has been reduced, because the need for instrumental delivery has fallen. Risk of birth injury declines when babies are born by propulsion, rather than by traction. Trauma is discussed as a separate item in Chapter 14. (See also *Tables* 4 and 5.)

Summary

No overall plan of management for labour can possibly be successful unless it starts from the premise that primigravidae and multigravidae are radically different creatures in almost every material respect. Inefficient uterine action is far the most common complication of childbirth; this is the reason why long and difficult labour occurs so much more often in primigravidae. The parous uterus, on the other hand, is a highly efficient organ; whenever labour proves troublesome in a multigravida the explanation should be sought elsewhere, beginning with obstruction.

One of the fundamental truths in clinical obstetrics is that the primigravid uterus is virtually immune to rupture whether or not oxytocin is used. The primigravida and her child are far more likely to have trauma inflicted on them by manipulation because of the greater need for instrumental delivery. Finally, probably the most pervasive error in the whole gamut of obstetrics is the practice of extrapolating from a first to a second labour. This results in treating last year's diseases. There is virtually no connection.

2: Induction v Acceleration

Just as there are fundamental differences between a first and a subsequent birth, there are fundamental differences between induction and acceleration. There exists a quite remarkable degree of confusion between these two procedures, despite the fact that a clear appreciation of the essential differences is a prerequisite to a rational approach to management of labour.

Failure to make a sufficiently sharp distinction between an attempt to interrupt the natural course of pregnancy, on the one hand, and to augment the course of labour – as a physiological process which has already begun – on the other hand, has misled doctors, nurses and mothers into the vague assumption that induction and acceleration are somehow extensions of the same procedure, merging imperceptibly into each other. This confusion stems mainly from the fact that membranes are ruptured artificially and oxytocin is infused in both instances. The logic of this position is comparable to a conclusion that no distinction need be drawn between diseases so totally dissimilar as amoebic dysentery and trichomonal vaginitis, because the therapeutic agent, metronidazole, is identical.

Duration of stress

Induction has the direct opposite effect to acceleration because induction extends the period of stress to which a woman is exposed – by the length of time which elapses before labour begins. As the main purpose of acceleration is to limit the period of stress to which a woman in labour is exposed, there is an obvious need to examine very closely indeed, all aspects of a procedure which has precisely the opposite result.

Diagnosis of labour

The diagnosis of labour is often obfuscated, hopelessly, by induction. The explanation for this is that artificial rupture of membranes is performed as part of the procedure and painful uterine contractions are stimulated with oxytocin. Even in normal circumstances painful uterine contractions are not reliable evidence of labour, but when they occur in response to oxytocin they must be regarded with even greater suspicion. Pains caused by oxytocin are very likely to cease should the infusion be withdrawn. Therefore, it is a mistake to base a diagnosis of labour on evidence of painful uterine contractions, supported by a 'show' or ruptured membranes, as recommended in spontaneous labour. The diagnosis of labour in a case of induction must rest on dilatation of cervix alone. The result is that it is well-nigh impossible to state at which point in time, if indeed ever, induction ends and labour begins. The critical importance of a correct initial diagnosis in overall management of labour, is discussed at some length in Chapter 5. There it is stated that diagnosis is the single most important item in terms of management and, furthermore, that whenever the diagnosis is wrong every action which follows is likely to compound the error. Nowhere is this more clearly apparent than in cases of induction.

Operative intervention

There is a sharp increase in the rate of surgical intervention in cases of induction. However, caesarean sections performed after induction are more often than not attributed to complications of labour, such as inefficient uterine action, cephalopelvic disproportion or occipitoposterior position, when the reality is that labour has not even started. The explanation is to be found in the mistaken belief that labour begins when a woman on oxytocin complains of painful uterine contractions. Alternatively, caesarean sections performed after induction are attributed to the indications for which the inductions were undertaken, such as pre-eclampsia or prolonged pregnancy, although these indications may seldom bear close scrutiny and would rarely, of themselves, justify caesarean section. There is a natural reluctance to acknowledge the plain truth: that caesarean section is required to retrieve a situation which stems from medical intervention, especially when the indication for this intervention lacks genuine substance.

Favourable comparisons are sometimes made between caesarean section rates in cases in which labour is induced and in cases in which labour is not induced. Invariably, these are false because they do not compare like with like. Whereas elective caesarean sections are included amongst cases not induced, a decision to induce labour is taken in the expectation of vaginal delivery. It follows that the caesarean section rate in induced cases should be considerably lower than in cases not induced; any discrepancy should be attributed to the procedure itself and separately recorded under the title 'failed induction'.

The operative vaginal delivery rate is also higher following induction. In addition, forceps are more often applied soon after full dilatation has been achieved because of the extended period of stress to which the woman has been exposed, and for this reason rotation is more likely to be required. Acceleration of labour, by way of contrast, reduces the rate of operative intervention because, labours being shorter, mothers are more likely to effect spontaneous delivery.

Analgesia

There is a sharp increase in demand for pain relief in cases of induction. This is reflected in the dosage of drugs used and in the number of epidurals requested. The increase in demand for analgesia is a measure of the increase in intensity and duration of stress imposed. A surfeit of drugs introduces further extraneous problems which are discussed in later chapters. Acceleration of labour, on the other hand, reduces demand for analgesia because labour has already begun before the need arises and because steps are then taken to ensure that delivery occurs within a reasonable timescale.

Effects on others

A high rate of induction subjects not only those mothers who are involved directly to a period of stress which is prolonged artificially; the adverse effects extend to encompass all women in labour. A high rate of induction has an important indirect bearing on others because the limited resources of a delivery unit – especially the human resources – are dissipated in caring for women who are not in labour. This dilution of personal attention, which is a cornerstone of good management, affects everyone; it is at complete variance with the concept of intensive care. It seems a strange paradox of contemporary delivery unit practice that women who are not in labour should receive more attention, and for a longer time, than women who are in labour.

Time and place

To ensure that the sharp distinction between induction and acceleration is rigidly maintained, induction is undertaken as an elective procedure at a fixed time of day in this hospital. Emergency inductions are not permitted. Moreover, artificial rupture of membranes is performed in a special location and the patient returns to the antenatal ward to await the onset of labour. A diagnosis of labour is mandatory before amniotomy can be performed or oxytocin be infused in the delivery unit. Hence, time and place are used to reinforce the message. This ensures that clear decisions are made, especially in respect of diagnosis of labour, before any form of intervention is allowed. The rationale is comparable to the use of coloured charts to differentiate between primigravidae and multigravidae, as described in the previous chapter. Induction of labour and acceleration of labour are discussed as separate issues in Chapters 8 and 24.

Summary

Induction has numerous adverse effects on the outcome of labour. Emotional and physical stress are both increased. The diagnosis of labour is hopelessly confused. Operative intervention rates are inflated. There is greater demand for analgesia. The quality of care extended to all mothers is diluted. As this constitutes a formidable list, cases of induction should be reported separately so that the full impact of this commonplace intervention can be clearly seen.

3: Malpresentations, Malformation, Twins

The third fundamental distinction which must be drawn before labour can be discussed in a rational manner, is between management of labour and treatment of obstetrical abnormalities. The present treatise, on management of labour, is confined to cases in which there is a single fetus, a vertex presentation and a normal head. Obstetrical abnormalities, particularly those which implicate the fetus directly, are specifically excluded from consideration because, inter alia, these may cause obstruction during labour, thus placing the fetus and sometimes even the mother at risk. Treatment of obstetrical abnormalities, which include malpresentations, hydrocephalus and twins, is discussed at length in standard textbooks where very little attention is paid to management of labour as a distinct entity. These topics are as much outside the scope of the present treatise as are obstetrical abnormalities which affect the mother more directly, for example eclampsia or haemorrhage.

A brief outline of the general approach to treatment of malpresentations, relevant malformation and twins, in this hospital, is given in this chapter. All subsequent chapters are written on the clear assumption that definitive steps have been taken to exclude these conditions beforehand. Nonetheless, all admissions are included in the final statistics.

Breech and face

The hazards of breech delivery are confined to the child, virtually the only danger to the mother is through obstetrical intervention. The approach to management of breech presentation in labour is entirely pragmatic. Vaginal delivery is preferred whenever this can be accomplished without any form of obstetrical intervention. Caesarean section is the only treatment allowed, whether the need should arise during the first or the second stage of labour. Oxytocin is not used to accelerate slow progress in breech presentation. X-ray pelvimetry is not practised because size and shape of pelvis are not factors taken into account in deciding the mode of delivery.

The approach to face presentation is along similar lines. Vaginal delivery is preferred whenever this can be accomplished without any form of obstetrical intervention. Caesarean section is the only treatment allowed. Oxytocin is not used to accelerate slow progress in face presentation.

Brow and shoulder

Brow presentation and shoulder presentation – the latter a rare occurrence in primigravidae – are always treated by caesarean section. These are two of the most notable causes of obstructed labour, which can so easily lead to rupture of uterus in multigravidae. Hence, brow presentation and shoulder presentation differ from breech presentation and face presentation in that they also place the life of the mother at risk. Treatment of malpresentations by corrective manipulation is not practised in this hospital. Oxytocin is not used.

Hydrocephalus

The only malformation likely to cause obstruction is hydrocephalus. This is the third notable cause of obstructed labour which is likely to lead to rupture of uterus in multigravidae. The condition is usually treated by simple aspiration through a spinal needle, sometimes through the mother's abdomen, and labour is allowed to proceed. Oxytocin is not used.

Twins

Twins are regarded as an obstetrical abnormality, mainly because the second twin is exposed to special hazards, even during the course of normal labour. The second twin may suffer the effects of hypoxia because, not being so readily accessible, it cannot be equally well supervised. Not infrequently, the second twin may be a victim of chronic placental insufficiency with retarded growth, resorption of liquor and passage of meconium, none of which is suspected until the membranes rupture after the first twin is safely born. This may be too late to take effective action. Furthermore, the second twin may become misplaced, typically as a shoulder presentation, after the birth of the first twin. Slow progress in twins is treated, invariably, by caesarean section. Oxytocin is not used.

Obstruction

Notwithstanding the fact that detection of malpresentations, relevant malformation and twins is an integral part of antenatal care, and that independent assessment at the point of admission is likewise mandatory, the final responsibility rests squarely on the person who makes the decision to use oxytocin to ensure that these named complications have been excluded in each case. The person who prescribes oxytocin for a woman in labour should be required to place the following items on permanent record: that the vertex presents, that the head is normal and that there is a single fetus. However, in practice, it is in multigravidae only that malpresentations and malformation present a serious threat to the mother, because it is in multigravidae only that obstruction is likely to lead to rupture of uterus, whether or not oxytocin is, mistakenly, used. The reason why oxytocin should be used with extreme caution, if ever, in multigravidae, is that the parous uterus is highly vulnerable in this regard. This is certainly not true in primigravidae. Inadvertently, over time, oxytocin has been given mistakenly to primigravidae with obstructed labour caused by malpresentations and malformation, but without untoward effect. This, of course, is freely acknowledged as a culpable error.

The three classical components of abnormal labour – inefficient uterine action, occipitoposterior position and cephalopelvic disproportion – are not classified as obstetrical abnormalities. These are regarded as clinical aberrations which arise in normal cases after admission to hospital. This is a point of great practical importance because there are many who practice obstetrics in the steadfast belief that cephalopelvic disproportion is an obstetrical abnormality which can be detected before labour begins. This results in many elective caesarean sections which are quite unnecessary and which, moreover, are wrongly reported as examples of cephalopelvic disproportion.

Summary

Every discourse on the subject of labour should be confined strictly to cases in which the vertex presents, the head is normal and there is a single fetus. The subject should not be confused by the introduction of obstetrical abnormalities, especially those which implicate the fetus as a cause of obstruction. This is a common mistake.

There is a grave obligation on the person responsible to ensure that malpresentations, hydrocephalus and twins have all been excluded before oxytocin is authorised. Obstructed labour should be recognised as a definitive clinical entity which is completely different from cephalopelvic disproportion. This distinction has particular relevance to multigravidae, in whom obstructed labour is far the most common cause of rupture of the intact uterus.

4: Duration of Labour

It would be difficult indeed to exaggerate the beneficial effects of an accurate working definition of duration of labour on everyday clinical practice, since failure to define what is clearly one of the basic parameters of obstetrics has been a major obstacle to improvements in management, for many years.[2]

Definition

In this hospital, duration of labour is defined as the number of hours a woman spends in the delivery unit, from the point of her admission until the time her baby is born. No allowance is made for time spent in labour at home. Speculation on the number of hours a woman may have been in labour before she chose to admit herself to hospital is a futile exercise. This is an argument which cannot be resolved satisfactorily and which, in any event, has no relevance to subsequent management. Incidentally, the third stage of labour is not included in this definition.

There are four reasons why duration of labour is so defined:

- Time of admission is a maternal decision.
- Professional responsibility begins when a woman elects to place herself in care.
- Duration can be recorded accurately for purposes of comparison.
- Mothers themselves tend to recall duration of labour in this manner.

Effectively, overall duration of labour is determined by the length of the first stage, because the number of hours taken for the cervix to dilate represents some 90% of the entire birth process. The second stage is short, by comparison, and contributes little to the overall problem of prolonged labour.

This definition of duration applies, equally, when a woman who is not in labour remains in the delivery unit for whatever reason. Hence, duration of labour in the case of a woman admitted for induction is likewise recorded as hours spent in the delivery unit, because this is the realistic measure of stress to which she is exposed. Although it is not possible to say at what point induction ends and labour begins, the procedure itself exposes the woman to the same pressures as if she were in labour for all of the time. The definition still applies even when induction fails and resort is made to caesarean section. Similarly, when a woman is retained in the delivery unit in error because of a wrong diagnosis of labour, duration is nonetheless recorded from the time of admission.

This means that duration of labour is entered for some women who are recognised in retrospect as not having been in labour at all. Such anomalies demonstrate the extent to which duration of labour is synonymous with time spent in the delivery unit of this hospital.

Advantages of short labour

The mean duration of first labour – without any form of medical intervention – is somewhat less than 6 hours in our experience. In general, women tolerate stress of this duration very well, and provided they have a reasonable understanding of the birth process and are not left alone for an instant, they require little in the way of analgesia and usually succeed in delivering themselves.

To the mother

The impact of labour must be evaluated as much in emotional as in physical terms. Both are more closely related to the number of hours spent in a delivery unit than to any other objective measurement. Although some women are already unduly perturbed at the point of admission, while others remain apparently unmoved after many hours have passed, most fall somewhere between the two extremes. The morale of the average woman begins to deteriorate perceptibly after 6 hours. After 12 hours the deterioration accelerates rapidly – in geometric rather than arithmetic progression almost – until, eventually, a stage is reached at which an adult woman is reduced to pleading for deliverance, unless she is rendered semi-conscious with drugs or lulled into a false sense of security with epidural anaesthesia. It cannot be emphasised too strongly that the profound emotional disturbance caused by prolonged labour may endure a lifetime. Consequently, no woman should be permitted to continue long enough in labour to need more than two standard doses of analgesia, by whatever route. Exogenous influences, other than time, which have a significant bearing on the emotional equilibrium of women in labour are: good antenatal education, continuous personal attention, and constructive use of drugs to relieve pain. These items are discussed in later chapters.

To the enormously important, if somewhat less tangible, emotional benefits must be added the physical benefits of short labour. Nowadays, no one should be permitted to continue nearly long enough in labour to require treatment for dehydration, ketosis or salt depletion. There is virtually no possibility of these disturbances arising within a strict timescale of 12 hours. These considerations assume even greater relevance in tropical climates where changes of this nature can occur so much more rapidly. There are also the noteworthy advantages of a lesser need for surgical intervention (caesarean section during the first stage and rotational forceps during the second stage), simply because fit mothers are better able to deliver themselves. Lastly, there is a greatly reduced demand for analgesic drugs, which means that mothers who are fully conscious retain ultimate control.

To the child

Duration of labour is equally important for the child. A fetus is exposed to the risk of hypoxia, mainly in the first stage, and of trauma, mainly in the second stage. There is especially close correlation between trauma and duration because long labours frequently end in difficult forceps extractions. In times past, the medical approach to prolonged labour was based on full dilatation of cervix as the natural line of demarcation between abdominal and vaginal delivery. The primary aim was to sustain the mother and, through her, hopefully, the baby, until full dilatation was reached. Full dilatation became an end in itself, and when this milestone was achieved the ordeal was brought to a speedy, and often forcible, conclusion. This meant that forceps were applied before the head could descend to the level at which rotation into the anterior position naturally occurs. Not infrequently, serious trauma was inflicted in the process. The circle of confusion was complete when the difficult manoeuvre, and consequent trauma were interpreted as evidence that prolonged labour, or dystocia, is a common expression of cephalopelvic disproportion. Emphatically, this is not so.

To the staff

Duration of labour is a matter which affects professional staff hardly less profoundly. A shared sense of impotence in the face of widespread physical suffering, and even moral degradation, frequently colours the attitude of nurses and doctors from their early student days. Those who subsequently choose to specialise react in different ways: obstetricians tend to avoid the delivery unit as much as possible, while midwives tend to resort to excessive use of analgesia to alleviate otherwise intolerable stress. Control of duration of labour is almost as important for staff as it is for mothers and babies.

To the administrators

Duration of labour is a matter of utmost practical importance to administrators too, because the delivery unit constitutes the bottleneck in a maternity service through which all the consumers must pass. The result is that it is not possible to plan maternity hospital accommodation, or to allocate professional staff on a rational basis, unless the number of consumer hours to be serviced can be calculated in advance. Here is a prime example of the application of principles of cost efficiency in contemporary medical planning, where good medicine and sound economics are seen to complement each other. Nowhere is this seen to better advantage than in a modern, efficient intensive care delivery unit.

Conclusion

Prolonged labour, in this hospital, was defined as 36 hours in 1963, reduced to 24 hours in 1968 and, finally, to 12 hours in 1972. A formal decision was taken on 1 January 1972 to restrict the duration of labour to 12 hours. After that date, no provision was made on the official record for labour to last a longer time. The result is a well established policy, of which all expectant mothers are fully aware: not to expose anyone to the stress of labour for more than 12 hours. Meanwhile, in excess of 150,000 babies have been born and every mother not close to an easy vaginal delivery after 12 hours has been submitted to caesarean section. Contrary to reasonable expectations, this practice did not lead to any significant increase in the incidence of caesarean section; what appeared likely to be lost on the swings has been more than recovered on the roundabouts. The wider implications of the consistently low incidence of caesarean section as compared to the startling increase in most other centres over the same period are considered in Chapter 27.

Summary

Duration is the kernel of the problem of labour management. More than any other objective measurement, duration determines the impact of childbirth, particularly on mothers, but also on babies, and on those who care for both of them. Duration of labour should be equated with hours spent in a delivery unit. The ability to restrict duration without extending the use of caesarean section represents a notable advance in contemporary obstetric practice.

Other benefits of limited duration include total abolition of dehydration, ketosis and salt depletion, and dramatic reduction in demand for analgesia. There is a decline in the need for instrumental vaginal delivery, especially rotational forceps, because, given labour of short duration, women are much better able to cope and, eventually, to deliver themselves.

Finally, duration is essentially a problem of first labour.

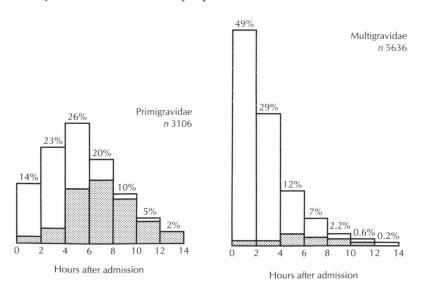

Figure 1. Duration of labour from time of admission to delivery unit. Shaded areas represent the proportion who received oxytocin: multigravidae include first vaginal deliveries after previous caesarean section.[3]

5: Diagnosis of Labour

The most important single item in the overall conduct of labour is diagnosis. When the initial diagnosis is wrong, all subsequent management is likely to be wrong too. The unfortunate consequences are to be seen almost daily in our delivery units, although these are seldom recognised for what they are. In medical circles there is an almost universal failure to appreciate that the diagnosis of labour represents a genuine problem. This has led to the altogether anomalous situation in which the fundamental decision, on which all subsequent management is based, is surrendered to mothers. Uniquely, an expectant mother admits herself to a maternity hospital, with the result that she tends to dictate her own treatment. This method of procedure, which leaves the initiative in the hands of 'patients', has no parallel in other branches of medicine.[4]

Doctors and midwives are noticeably vague whenever questions are asked about diagnosis of labour. Hence it should come as no surprise that mothers, especially primigravidae who lack previous experience, should sometimes be mistaken and admit themselves to hospital in error. Perhaps the most surprising feature is not that mothers are sometimes wrong, but that they are usually right. There are very few maternity centres where any serious attention is devoted to the diagnosis of labour. The general assumption is that no such problem exists, because women are naturally endowed with an unerring instinct that enables them to make a correct decision in these matters. The subject is not discussed at any length in textbooks and is evaded in medical publications, where only cases said to be in 'established' labour – because the cervix is well dilated – are included in scientific reports. The common practice is to resort to the convenient device of making a retrospective decision that a woman has been in labour after her baby is born. In everyday practice, however, decisions must be prospective; medicine in real life does not afford the luxury of wisdom after the event. An essential difference between the theory and the practice of obstetrics is that the doctor or, more likely, the midwife does not enjoy the benefit of hindsight when an agitated primigravida presents herself at a delivery unit late at night because she thinks she is in labour. A firm decision is required in these circumstances. Equivocal terms such as false labour, latent labour or labour not established, serve only as stratagems to relieve the doctor or midwife of the onus of having to make this decision. Such terms have no real meaning. The effect, however, is to pass the responsibility for the diagnosis of labour back to the patient, where it certainly does not belong. Most errors in management of labour result from decisions avoided, rather than from decisions wrongly made. This dictum applies with particular force to the initial diagnosis.

First step

The first step in management of labour is to confirm, or deny, the pre-sumptive diagnosis which has been made by the mother prior to admission. There are strict instructions to this effect in this hospital, and these instructions must be put into practice not later than one hour after admission. The midwife in charge of the delivery unit is nominated as the person directly responsible. The official chart, or partograph, is designed in such a manner as to ensure that the evidence on which her decision is based is committed to permanent record. The terms are both simple and explicit. This evidence is located in the most prominent position. Thus, a prospective diagnosis of labour is made in every case admitted and the evidence on which this was based remains available, even when the individual concerned has gone off duty. (See *Graph 3*.)

Meanwhile, no treatment whatsoever is permitted until a firm diagnosis of labour is made, because treatment of any kind almost certainly commits a woman to delivery, whether or not she is in labour. Naturally, whenever a woman's presumptive diagnosis of labour is not accepted by staff she deserves an adequate explanation, couched in simple language which she can understand. The explanation given in this hospital is a paraphrase of what is written here; it is almost universally well received. Then, the woman is transferred to an antenatal ward where she is invariably retained until the next day. A woman who is adjudged not to be in labour is not retained in the precincts of the delivery unit for one moment longer than is absolutely necessary, and never for longer than one hour, but neither is she allowed to return home, lest the passage of time should prove her diagnosis to have been correct which, inevitably, will sometimes transpire.

Pains

A woman's diagnosis of labour is based on the subjective element of pain. Pain is such a constant feature that without pain the question of labour simply does not arise. However, not every woman who complains of pain is necessarily in labour, although late in pregnancy this is by no means an unreasonable assumption. The nature and the distribution of the particular pain may be so uncharacteristic that it bears no resemblance whatever to labour, in which case it can be discounted readily by an experienced observer. Alternatively, the pain may be so characteristic – intermittent, symmetrical and coincident with uterine contractions – that it can make for a much more difficult decision.

There is a popular misconception, prevalent even in professional circles, that pain which coincides with uterine contractions provides conclusive evidence of labour. This is an elementary mistake. A doctor or midwife with hand on abdomen to confirm that a woman winces as her uterus contracts needs to appreciate that Braxton Hicks contractions, which are a normal feature of late pregnancy, increase both in strength and frequency as term approaches and, furthermore, that they can cause considerable discomfort when the threshold for pain is low. Pain of this nature cannot be distinguished from pain of labour because of the common origin. The threshold for pain is reduced mainly through anxiety, which is most likely to occur late at night, especially when a woman is alone, or resides at a considerable distance from the hospital service. Understandably a woman who fears that she may arrive too late tends to travel too early. These are salient factors which should be taken into account when a diagnosis of labour is under consideration.

An air of uncertainty at the point of admission compounds the problem still further, because the woman quickly senses that the experts from whom she had a right to expect guidance cannot even recognise labour! Instead of firm direction she meets with evasion, which undermines her confidence even more. As anxiety increases the pain worsens. Unfortunately, staff are wont to respond with analgesic drugs; these have the indirect effect of committing the woman to delivery. Therefore, it must be made crystal clear that painful uterine contractions alone do not warrant a professional diagnosis of labour. Painful uterine contractions need to be supported by evidence of a more objective nature before a professional diagnosis of labour can be upheld.

Effacement and dilatation

Diagnosis of labour presents no problem whenever painful uterine contractions are combined with dilatation of cervix, since the very essence of labour is opening of the neck of the womb. A woman who enters hospital with her cervix well dilated is not only surely in labour, she can be expected to proceed rapidly and deliver normally within a matter of a few hours. The extent of dilatation of cervix at the point of admission is a clear indication of the efficiency of uterine action: it is not, as often supposed, a reflection of the number of hours spent in labour at home. Reports in medical journals which are confined to cases in which labour is said to be 'established' do not merely evade the fundamental problem of diagnosis, but also exclude from consideration the very cases which are likely to cause problems in subsequent management. As these are the women who suffer from inefficient uterine action, such selective reporting can be very misleading.

Since dilatation of cervix represents the sole conclusive evidence of labour, it is clearly essential that this term be accurately defined. Of necessity, this entails definition of the term effacement also, because the two events are so closely related and frequently confused. Chapter 26 is devoted to consideration of these two critical events in greater detail. Meanwhile, the term effacement refers to incorporation of the cervical canal into the lower uterine segment. This proceeds from above downwards, that is from the internal os to the external os. The process may either occur late in pregnancy or be delayed until labour begins. Dilatation, on the other hand, refers only to the external os. This does not begin to open until the entire length of the canal has been eliminated, at which point effacement is complete. As this marks a point of transition, to speak in terms of dilatation before effacement is complete involves a direct contradiction of terms.

The external os is seldom so tightly closed that it does not admit a fingertip long before labour is due to begin. This can be a source of confusion when a fingertip is equated with one centimetre on the notional metric scale used to express the extent of dilatation of cervix during labour. Effacement is the feature which serves to distinguish between the cervix which passively admits a fingertip, and the cervix which is actively dilated to the extent of one centimetre in labour. A diagnosis of labour is made when a woman admits herself to this hospital with painful uterine contractions and the cervix is found to be effaced completely on pelvic examination. Such a woman is retained in the delivery unit and therefore committed to delivery within 12 hours.

With regard to diagnosis of labour, the problem cases are to be found among the considerable number of women who admit themselves to hospital with painful uterine contractions but in whom the cervix is not completely effaced. In these circumstances, objective evidence of a different order must be sought. A 'show' or spontaneous rupture of membranes represent the alternatives. These simple signs provide invaluable aids to diagnosis when the cervix is not completely effaced.

'Show'

A 'show', or blood-stained plug of mucus, passed early – often before effacement is complete and dilatation can therefore begin – is easily recognised by mothers and staff alike and, consequently, has an important role to play in the diagnosis of labour. Although not conclusive, a show affords presumptive evidence of dynamic change in the condition of the cervix which is sufficient to cause the plug of mucus to be extruded.

A diagnosis of labour is made in this hospital when subjective evidence of pain is supported by objective evidence of a show, even though the cervix may not be effaced, let alone dilated. A woman with painful uterine contractions and a show is retained in the delivery unit and, consequently, committed to delivery within 12 hours, without regard to the condition of her cervix. An exception is sometimes made in the case of a woman who is less than 37 weeks gestation, in the somewhat vain hope that labour may be somehow averted. A show has already occurred in approximately 70% of women who admit themselves to this hospital in the belief that they are in labour.

Naturally, a show without painful uterine contractions does not warrant the same interpretation. A show in such circumstances is recorded as an unsubstantial antepartum haemorrhage, and the woman is transferred to the antenatal ward. A show which follows vaginal examination is regarded as an artefact, about which anyone exposed to the procedure is given prior notice.

Ruptured membranes

Spontaneous rupture of membranes is accepted as even stronger pre-sumptive evidence of labour than a show. A diagnosis of labour is made when a woman admits herself to this hospital with painful uterine contractions supported by spontaneous rupture of membranes. She is retained in the delivery unit and, therefore, committed to delivery within 12 hours, without regard to the condition of her cervix. Spontaneous rupture of membranes has already occurred in approximately 30% of women who admit themselves to this hospital in the belief that they are in labour.

Similarly, spontaneous rupture of membranes alone does not warrant a diagnosis of labour. Membranes not infrequently rupture several weeks before labour eventually begins. A woman with spontaneous rupture of membranes but no painful uterine contractions is transferred to the antenatal ward. Even when the gestation in question exceeds 42 weeks a decision as to whether to attempt to induce labour with oxytocin must be deferred until the next day. Induction is permitted only as an elective procedure; emergency inductions are not allowed. This strict rule serves to maintain the sharp distinction between acceleration of labour which has already begun and initiation of labour which has not yet started. Hence, the challenge of diagnosis of labour must be confronted at every step along the way. In the event of a woman with spontaneous rupture of membranes returning to the delivery unit within a few hours, it is not always concluded that the initial decision was necessarily wrong. More likely, the correct explanation in this situation is that meanwhile the woman has, so to speak, induced labour on herself. Rupture of membranes, whether it be artificial or spontaneous, is an effective method of initiating labour.

Vaginal examination is strictly prohibited if there is any likelihood that a woman admitted with spontaneous rupture of membranes may not be in labour. This is to prevent the introduction of infection which could gravely prejudice the final outcome. A casual vaginal examination performed on a woman with ruptured membranes effectively commits her to delivery whether or not she is in labour. Eventually this may require an unnecessary caesarean section. Consequently, routine performance of vaginal examination at the point of admission to a delivery unit is indicative of a lack of foresight in this regard. There are additional grounds for this reservation when gestation is less than 37 weeks, and it seems desirable that delivery be postponed as long as possible in the interest of maturity.

A show and spontaneous rupture of membranes count as two independent signs of labour when the show appears first, but as one sign only when the membranes rupture first, because the significance of a show is vitiated by prior rupture of membranes.

Errors in diagnosis

An error in diagnosis of labour can be made either way.

A woman's diagnosis of labour may be accepted, in which case she is retained in the delivery unit and exposed to the manifold pressures of that particular environment. Inevitably, her morale begins to crumble and her physical condition eventually deteriorates as time passes and no progress is made. The problem is compounded by analgesic drugs or epidural block, and possibly oxytocin, until a point is reached at which there is no option but to terminate her ordeal by resort to caesarean section. The record will doubtless show that caesarean section was performed for maternal or fetal distress caused by prolonged labour, whereas the truth of the matter is that the initial diagnosis of labour was incorrect: a state of labour never existed. The first occasion when such a woman is seen by the consultant obstetrician may well be when he is to perform the operation. The clinical history available at this juncture is likely, at best, to be secondhand. Now, it is frequently impossible to identify the person who made the critical decision, much less review the evidence on which that decision was based. In practice these questions are seldom even asked, simply because their significance is not widely appreciated.

Alternatively, a woman's diagnosis of labour may be rejected by staff, in which case she is transferred to the antenatal ward, perhaps to return a short time later well advanced in labour. This is not a serious mistake, provided that she is not sent home. To guard against this eventuality, every woman who admits herself to this hospital because she thinks she is in labour is retained until the following day.

Of course, it must be openly acknowledged that no matter how much careful attention is paid to the diagnosis of labour, subsequent events will sometimes prove it wrong, because it is just not humanly possible to make a correct decision in every case. No method of diagnosis is foolproof. The aim should be to reduce the number of errors to a minimum, while simultaneously operating a fail-safe procedure which ensures, insofar as possible, that whenever an error does occur it can be retrieved in good time, as follows.

The woman who is retained in the delivery unit in error

Here, failure of the cervix to respond to oxytocin, which will be used at some stage to rectify slow progress, should quickly raise the suspicion that a mistake has been made. Treatment should be stopped before the point of no return is reached. The true position should be explained to the mother, in intelligible terms, and she should be transferred to the antenatal ward. This woman is likely to return some hours later and proceed to deliver rapidly, because on this occasion she is in labour. The ability to retrieve an admittedly difficult situation depends partly on the sense of trust which the mother places in the staff and partly on the confidence that the staff have in themselves; self confidence and mutual respect permit mistakes to be acknowledged and freely discussed. These characteristics are, in themselves, very closely related to overall standards of practice in a delivery unit. However, some mothers do become so distressed by the unfortunate experience that it is not possible to return to the original position: in this event, caesarean section is the only solution. But the fact remains that the true state of affairs in these cases is seldom recognised. Approximately 10% of women who admit themselves to this hospital under the impression that they are in labour are mistaken. It is a matter of utmost importance that these individuals be identified before they find themselves on a production line from which there is but one escape route: caesarean section, and that after much anguish.

The woman who is transferred to an antenatal ward because her diagnosis of labour is not accepted

She is not allowed home under any circumstances, until she is formally discharged on the following day. This precaution eliminates the possible embarrassment of giving birth in transit. Incidentally, a woman with painful uterine contractions who returns to the delivery unit before discharge is presumed to have been in labour at first admission.

Diagnosis after induction

Finally, a note about induction. Anyone who is genuinely concerned about the quality of care in labour must look very closely indeed at the practice of induction, a subject about which more is written in Chapter 24. In the present context, it cannot be emphasised too strongly that a procedure which includes artificial rupture of membranes and infusion of oxytocin, plays havoc with the diagnosis of labour. Oxytocin causes painful uterine contractions, whether or not a woman is in labour; this is a vivid example of the commonplace fallacy of basing a diagnosis of labour on painful uterine contractions alone. In the course of induction the significance of painful uterine contractions, a show, and ruptured membranes are all nullified. Hence the diagnosis of labour in a case of induction rests solely on dilatation of cervix. The fact that this is not generally appreciated leads to widespread confusion about when induction ends and labour begins. This provides the opportunity of attributing an adverse outcome in such cases to a complication of labour rather than to a failed induction, where it correctly belongs.

There is one other aspect of the problem of diagnosis of labour worthy of brief comment. This concerns claims made for treatment aimed at arresting the course of labour which has started prematurely. The credibility of these claims rests entirely on whether or not the subjects treated were actually in labour to begin with; that is, on the accuracy of the initial diagnosis. Advocates of this form of therapy tend to start from the premise that the diagnosis of labour is such a simple matter that it can be taken for granted. Needless to say, this is far from the truth. Such scant attention is paid to the problem of diagnosis of labour at term, that it may come as a surprise to find the ease with which it is made prematurely in publications advocating the benefits of tocolytic agents.[5]

Summary

Diagnosis is the single most important item in the whole conduct of labour. Significantly, this is the longest chapter in the book. As with every syndrome in clinical medicine, labour too must begin with a correct diagnosis; an incorrect diagnosis inevitably leads to inappropriate treatment. A clinical diagnosis must, of its nature, be prospective and a diagnosis of labour is, in effect, a positive decision to commit a woman to delivery. Clearly, a matter of such consequence should not be left to lay persons to decide.

Painful uterine contractions alone do not warrant a medical diagnosis of labour. Pains must be supported by a show, by spontaneous rupture of membranes, or by dilatation of cervix. Although dilatation of cervix represents the sole conclusive evidence of labour, in practice either a show or spontaneous rupture of membranes, combined with painful uterine contractions, affords sufficiently strong, albeit presumptive, evidence to commit a woman to delivery. Given the critical importance of dilatation of cervix, it is clearly imperative that the term should be accurately defined.

There are two common errors: first, treatment may be initiated on the basis of painful uterine contractions unsupported by other evidence of labour; and second, treatment may be withheld although painful uterine contractions are supported by a show or spontaneous rupture of membranes, because the cervix is not dilated. The possibility that subsequent events may show the initial diagnosis to have been incorrect should be kept constantly in mind.

6: Progress: First Stage

After the diagnosis of labour has been confirmed, the next important item in management is to monitor progress, at short and regular intervals, especially in the early hours. Progress during the first stage of labour is measured exclusively in terms of dilatation of cervix because the sole function of uterine action during the first stage of labour is to open the exit from the womb sufficiently to allow the baby's head to pass. The rate of dilatation of cervix is crucial because the duration of labour depends almost entirely on the duration of the first stage. This is true to the extent that the two are almost synonymous in everyday clinical practice. The first stage accounts for some 90% of the entire duration of labour in normal circumstances.

Descent of head certainly is not an appropriate measure of progress during the first stage of labour. There is no consistent relationship between dilatation of cervix and descent of head. Descent of head is the measure of progress appropriate to the second stage of labour. The sole function of uterine action during the second stage of labour is to propel the fetus along the birth canal.

Pelvic examination

Pelvic examination is performed at the point of admission, and repeated thereafter at regular intervals of one hour for the next three hours. Subsequent examinations are performed at the discretion of the examiner, but at intervals not longer than two hours. Successive examinations are performed by the same person, as far as possible, because there is as a considerable subjective element in interpretation. Dilatation of cervix is not susceptible to accurate measurement; consequently, this is one clinical situation where too many cooks will surely spoil the broth. The midwife in charge of the delivery unit is named as the person responsible for assessment of progress in this hospital, just as she is also responsible for diagnosis of labour. The subjective element in interpretation is most pronounced at times when changes of staff occur; this possibility should be kept always in mind because it has a practical bearing on management, where a false impression of secondary arrest in progress is easily created.

Vaginal examination is potentially dangerous when there is a possibility of ruptured membranes in a woman who may not be in labour. Examination in these circumstances commits a woman to delivery because of the risk of infection; this could result in the birth of a preterm infant, or in a caesarean section undertaken to retrieve iatrogenic disease. In this hospital, vaginal examination is discouraged when there is a possibility of ruptured membranes, unless a strong presumptive diagnosis of labour has already been made.

Cervical dilatation

The degree of dilatation of cervix is recorded on a simple graph and plotted against hours after admission. Full dilatation is equated with 10 cm because this is the approximate diameter of a newborn baby's head. The maximum time allotted is 10 hours. It follows that the slowest rate of dilatation acceptable is 1 cm each hour. The whole purpose of the graph is to relate progress to passage of time in a visual manner which is readily intelligible, even to a lay person. Selected illustrations are provided in Section II of this manual. The extent to which rate of progress dominates all other aspects of labour should be noted. Graphic records of labour are so often crammed with minute detail that the visual impact is lost completely; the result is that the main purpose of the exercise is defeated. Efforts to include every conceivable detail of every aspect of labour, whether relevant to the central issue or not, are, therefore, counterproductive.

A clear pattern of dilatation should have emerged at the end of three hours: on this basis it should be possible to predict the hour of delivery by simple linear projection in all but a few instances. Close attention to progress during the early hours of labour is the best insurance against difficulty later. The weight of emphasis currently placed on the first three hours of labour stands in sharp contrast with our previous practice, when no worthwhile medical decision was considered necessary until a woman had been in labour for several hours and complications had begun to threaten. Those belated decisions were concerned primarily with the rescue of mothers and babies from potentially dangerous predicaments which had developed over a protracted period of time, in normal cases, after admission to hospital. No serious thought was given to prevention.

Four hours is much too long to wait to discover that labour has not progressed since a previous examination and it is much too long to wait to discover that treatment prescribed to accelerate slow progress after a previous examination has not been successful. Prolonged labour is far more likely to occur where pelvic examination is performed at infrequent and irregular intervals; infrequent and irregular pelvic examinations encourage a tolerant attitude to prolonged labour.

An unsatisfactory rate of dilatation of cervix during the early hours of labour is a clear and unequivocal expression of inefficient uterine action. The defect should be corrected without undue delay. This pattern of dilatation has no relevance whatever to cephalopelvic disproportion, a false association which has given rise to a great deal of confusion in times past. Treatment of inefficient uterine action is discussed in Chapter 8, and illustrated in *Graphs 19* and *20*.

Communication

One of the main benefits to accrue from pelvic assessment at relatively short intervals is the ability to keep the mother regularly posted on the progress of events. Hopefully, it will have been explained to her before-hand, at antenatal classes, that the purpose of pelvic examination is to measure the speed at which the neck of her womb opens, because this effectively determines the length of her labour. In that case, she will already be familiar with the partograph. As time passes the result of each examination is conveyed directly to her by the examiner as it is being entered on the graph. As a lay person is not accustomed to think in terms of dilatation of cervix, but merely anxious to know when her baby will be born, attention is focused on the time scale. The need to be convinced that steady progress is being made, and to appreciate that there is a predictable end in sight, are matters of prime importance to the morale of all participants in the birth process.

The standard practice in this hospital is to inform every woman in labour of the projected time of her delivery as soon as a clear pattern of dilatation is established; this is seldom later than three hours after admission. Time of delivery is stated to within 30 minutes. At noon, the woman is told that her baby is expected at 4 o'clock in the afternoon, give or take a half hour. This information is updated after each examination. No examination is undertaken on a woman in labour without her direct involvement and in deference to her before, during and after the event. She must know the purpose of the examination and be the first to learn of the result. The onus rests squarely on the examiner to ensure that she genuinely understands the real meaning of what is being said. Platitudes, to the effect that 'all is well' or 'progress is as good as can be expected', are not tolerated. These inanities constitute an affront to the intelligence of women generally, and thus serve to undermine mutual confidence. Similarly, technical terms are strictly avoided. These are seen as a cloak for ignorance; an examiner who does not really comprehend the implications of the signs elicited is in no position to explain them to a third party and therefore retreats behind medical jargon.

Summary

The sole purpose of uterine action during the first stage of labour is to open the neck of the womb sufficiently to allow the baby's head to pass. Hence, dilatation of cervix is the only measure of progress appropriate to the first stage of labour. Dilatation of cervix proceeds on a straight line, the direction of which is evident within a few hours after admission. This makes it eminently feasible to predict the approximate time of delivery, or, alternately, to take prompt corrective action against the drift into prolonged labour. Regular pelvic assessment should be mandatory after each of the first three hours.

7: Progress: Second Stage

The second stage of labour begins at full dilatation. In practice, this means no part of the cervix is palpable at pelvic examination. For record purposes only, full dilatation is equated with 10 centimetres, because this is the approximate width of the mature fetal head. Progress in the second stage of labour is measured in terms of descent and, incidentally, rotation.

The contribution of the second stage to the total duration of labour is relatively small, because the second stage seldom lasts longer than two hours. The second stage of labour deserves particular attention because of the special risk of trauma. Although trauma is confined, virtually, to the second stage of labour, antecedent events are often highly relevant. With the notable exception of breech presentation, serious injury to the child is almost always associated with operative intervention to effect birth by traction, because the mother is unable, unwilling or, perhaps, not given the opportunity to deliver herself.

Such was the emphasis placed on full dilatation in previous times that it became generally accepted as the natural line of demarcation between abdominal and vaginal delivery. This is a serious fallacy, one fraught with gravest consequences. In practical terms, the second stage of labour is composed of two quite distinct phases: the first phase extends from full dilatation until the head reaches the pelvic floor, the second phase extends from then until the baby is born. These two phases are as different from each other as chalk is from cheese. The second stage of labour, in other words, is not a single entity.

Phase one

During phase one of the second stage of labour, the head is relatively high in the pelvis, the occiput is in the transverse diameter, the vagina is not stretched and there is no inclination on the part of the mother to push. Neither the mother nor her attendants are aware of any significant change, and the fact that the cervix has reached full dilatation would pass entirely without notice unless, perchance, a pelvic examination was performed at this juncture. This phase is but a natural extension of the first stage of labour and treatment should not differ in any way. A woman with no inclination to push should not be urged to do so. No attempt should be made to achieve vaginal delivery by traction, and whenever the need for urgent delivery arises this should be by caesarean section. In terms of management, therefore, full dilatation of cervix is an event of academic interest only. This reservation applies to the time element also, a subject discussed in the following paragraph.

Phase two

Phase two of the second stage of labour begins when the head impacts on the floor of the pelvis, an event which coincides with a dramatic change in the demeanour of the mother. Vaginal delivery is virtually assured at this point, and whenever the need for intervention arises the standard obstetric forceps, or ventouse, can be used. The duration of this phase must be restricted because of the exceptional physical strain to which both mother and child are subjected by the compulsive urge to push. This is where the time factor becomes a vital consideration. There is no corresponding need to restrict the duration of phase one, because the element of exceptional physical strain does not apply.

Some of the most potentially dangerous misunderstandings in current obstetric practice stem from failure to draw a sharp distinction between these two phases of the second stage of labour. The classical example is when forceps are applied as a matter of routine, simply because the cervix is known to be fully dilated for an arbitrary period of time. A difficult rotation is followed by strong traction to overcome soft tissue resistance. This leads to a diagnosis of cephalopelvic disproportion where none exists. The mother is exposed to the immediate risk of serious injury, and her future plans are prejudiced by prior committal to elective caesarean section on the basis of an incorrect interpretation of the sequence of events. Moreover, should the child die, and necropsy show evidence of trauma, or survive with brain damage, this is misinterpreted as further confirmation for the diagnosis of cephalopelvic disproportion.

Forceps

The conventional method of treatment of slow progress in the second stage of labour, is forceps extraction. Forceps are applied in three distinct clinical circumstances which are quite different from one another, as follows:

First, the instrument may be applied as soon as full dilatation is achieved after a long first stage of labour. The declared purpose is to bring the mothers' ordeal to a speedy conclusion, or to anticipate fetal distress based sometimes on slender evidence. This being phase one of the second stage, the head is still high in the transverse diameter of the pelvis. Delivery entails rotation, frequently with Kielland's forceps, followed by strong traction to overcome soft tissue resistance, because although the cervix is sufficiently dilated, the vagina is most certainly not. This manoeuvre is, arguably, the main source of serious injury to both mother and child in contemporary obstetrics. Perpetuation of the manoeuvre is based on the archaic proposition that full dilatation of cervix is the natural line of demarcation between abdominal and vaginal delivery. This situation must change. It must be recognised that a case of this nature would fare much better if full dilatation was never achieved. At least this would protect against misguided attempts at forcible vaginal delivery. It hardly needs to be said that the use of forceps, or ventouse, during the first stage of labour is indefensible in all circumstances.

Second, the instrument may be applied when uterine action fails, as a secondary phenomenon, after a normal first stage of labour. The head remains high, in the transverse position, because the driving force is inadequate. From the standpoint of vaginal delivery, the prospect is the same as in the previous paragraph: the woman remains stranded in phase one of the second stage of labour.

Third, the instrument may be applied after the head has reached the floor of the pelvis when, despite good uterine action, the mother is unable to overcome the formidable obstacle presented by the levator muscles through her own efforts. Not infrequently, this impasse arises because the mother is emotionally and physically exhausted after a long first stage, or mentally confused by a large dosage of drugs. She has, however, made the critical transition from phase one to phase two of the second stage of labour, to the point at which extraction with forceps or ventouse is a comparatively safe procedure. The vagina, as well as the cervix, is now dilated.

Oxytocin as alternative

Conventional methods of treatment in phase one of the second stage of labour offer a straight choice between caesarean section and difficult forceps extraction. Faced with these alternatives, preference should be for caesarean section, in the interest of all parties concerned.

There is, however, a third option available: oxytocin. The relatively common clinical problem described above provides one of the most impressive examples of the constructive use of oxytocin across the whole of obstetrics. An oxytocin infusion begun in the second stage of labour restores normal uterine action; this causes the head to descend to the pelvic floor and also, hopefully, to rotate at that level. The result is that a difficult rotational forceps delivery is translated into an easy extraction, if not, indeed, a spontaneous delivery. There is no better practical illustration of one of the basic concepts of active management of labour: that delivery by propulsion is preferable, almost invariably, to delivery by traction. The intelligent use of oxytocin introduced in the second stage of labour has made an important contribution to reduction in the incidence of trauma, to both mothers and infants in this hospital in recent years. See *Table 5* and *Graph 17*.

Summary

Full dilatation of cervix is not the natural line of division between abdominal and vaginal delivery. The second stage of labour is composed of two distinct phases. The natural line of division between abdominal and vaginal delivery, comes at the end of phase one, when the head has descended to the floor of the pelvis, where rotation normally occurs. Vaginal delivery with forceps, or ventouse, should not be attempted simply because the case has entered the second stage; not only the cervix but also the vagina needs to be fully dilated.

Kielland's forceps has long ago been discarded from this hospital. There has been no consequent increase in the rate of caesarean section. The explanation, at least in part, lies in the use of oxytocin in the second stage. This novel procedure represents an important contribution to the conduct of labour, particularly where trauma is concerned.

8: Acceleration of Slow Labour

The most important decisions relating to management of labour are made during the first three hours. The decision to accelerate is one of these. Three hours after admission to a delivery unit, the course of labour should be set to the extent that it ought then be possible to predict the approximate time of delivery in all but a few instances. The ability to predict the time of delivery at this comparatively early stage is of inestimable value to all who are involved in the birth process.

Procedure

Circumstances dictate that the decision to accelerate progress – like the diagnosis of labour – must be made by a midwife, because midwives, unlike obstetricians, are physically present in the delivery unit at all times. Crucial decisions on management must not be allowed to go by default simply because women admit themselves in labour at inconvenient hours. The duty of the consultant obstetrician is to state clearly the basic rules of procedure and this should entail accepting responsibility for the result. Prolonged labour has been virtually eliminated from this hospital, mainly because the midwife in charge of the delivery unit knows precisely what to do, and when to do it. She knows, too, that no blame will attach to her in the event of an adverse outcome. This is a vital consideration, failing which no plan of action is likely to succeed. The procedure is outlined below.

First assessment

Progress is assessed, initially, at 1 hour after admission. Artificial rupture of membranes is now performed. Apart from the fact that the nature of the liquor provides material evidence of the fetal condition and, therefore, should be ascertained in every case, there are four additional reasons why the membranes are ruptured at this juncture:

- In the event of slow progress, rupture of membranes alone may be sufficient to accelerate. See *Graph 18*.
- Oxytocin is not permitted unless clear liquor is seen.
- Oxytocin may be ineffective with intact membranes.
- Theoretically, oxytocin may increase the risk of amniotic fluid infusion into the maternal circulation unless free drainage has been established.

Spontaneous rupture of membranes has already occurred in some 30% of women who admit themselves to this hospital in labour.

Second assessment

Progress is assessed for the second time at 2 hours after admission. An oxytocin infusion is started unless significant progress – one notional centimetre – has been made since the previous examination. The decision to use oxytocin is taken by the midwife in charge without reference to medical personnel.

The following conditions must be fulfilled:

- The mother must be nulliparous.
- The presentation must be vertex.
- The fetus must be single.
- The membranes must be ruptured and clear liquor seen.

Oxytocin is prohibited in parous women, in malpresentations and twins, when membranes are intact, or when meconium, or no liquor, is seen. The reasons for these exclusions are discussed elsewhere. Special attention is drawn to the fact that oxytocin may not be given to a parous woman without direction, in each individual case, by a senior member of medical staff, who must then assume immediate personal responsibility for all further conduct of the case. The decision to give oxytocin to a parous woman cannot be taken by a midwife or junior doctor, nor can they be held responsible for any subsequent mishap.

Third assessment

Progress is assessed for the third time at 3 hours after admission. A dramatic change is expected. Now it should be possible to predict full dilatation, and consequent delivery, from a linear projection on the partograph. See *Graph 11*.

Subsequent assessments

Further progress is assessed at intervals not exceeding two hours. In practice, the next examination is likely to be performed to confirm full dilatation, when the mother feels the urge to push.

This makes a total of five pelvic examinations in the course of an average labour: at admission to confirm the diagnosis of labour, at 1, 2 and 3 hours to monitor progress and, finally, before the mother is allowed to push.

Slow progress

In the most unlikely event of failure to respond to treatment with oxytocin for a period of one hour, there are two possible explanations to be considered. First, the woman may not be in labour because the initial diagnosis was wrong. Second, the forewaters may be intact despite the fact that liquor may have been seen to drain. Once again, acceleration must not be confused with induction, where oxytocin frequently proves ineffective. See *Graphs 21* and *22*.

Slow progress in labour is almost confined to women in whom the cervix is less than 2 cm dilated at time of admission. When the cervix is more than 2 cm dilated at time of admission there are few problems to be faced: diagnosis is easy, progress is rapid, and spontaneous delivery is likely to take place within a matter of hours. The extent to which the cervix is dilated at time of admission is an accurate reflection of the quality of uterine action; contrary to widespread belief, it bears little, if any, relationship to the number of hours a woman has spent in labour at home. Forty per cent of primigravidae deliver themselves within four hours of admission to this hospital. See *Table 8*.

Secondary arrest

In the much less likely event of secondary arrest in progress during the first stage of labour, when dilatation has been satisfactory in the early hours but comes to a virtual halt later, the same procedure is followed. Oxytocin is infused in a similar manner. Caesarean section is undertaken after one hour unless, meanwhile, normal progress has resumed. This unusual pattern of dilatation raises the question of cephalopelvic disproportion for the first time and the diagnosis is taken as confirmed should the pattern persist after uterine action has been restored.

Secondary arrest in progress may not occur until the second stage of labour when, after full dilatation has been achieved, the head does not descend. Failure of descent is the clinical manifestation of 'dystocia' during the second stage of labour and should be seen as the counterpart of failure to dilate during the first stage. The same procedure is followed: oxytocin is infused. The use of oxytocin during the second stage of labour is discussed in Chapter 7. See *Graph 24*.

Summary

Duration of labour is effectively determined by rate of dilatation of cervix, especially in the early hours; therefore, it is particularly important that dilatation be monitored during this critical period. This requires pelvic examination at regular intervals for the first three hours. A midwife is the only person in a position to conduct these examinations around the clock, and to make the decision to respond when progress is slow. To meet this commitment, she must have explicit instructions and she must enjoy the unqualified support of her medical colleagues. The uterus in labour is almost uniformly responsive to oxytocin provided the forewaters are ruptured. Oxytocin should not be given to parous women, at least without authorisation at the highest medical level on each occasion.

9: Oxytocin in Labour

Oxytocin is one of the most specific therapeutic agents available in medicine. Properly used, it can also be one of the safest. The therapeutic effect of oxytocin is to cause the cervix to dilate during the first stage, and the head to descend during the second stage. This sequential action is almost invariably achieved. Indeed, the effect of oxytocin is so predictable that when the cervix does not dilate during the first stage, by far the most likely explanation is that the woman is not in labour. Failure of the cervix to dilate in response to oxytocin constitutes a clear indication to review the diagnosis of labour, and here again it is necessary to emphasise the fundamental difference between induction of labour and acceleration of labour, because oxytocin is not nearly so predictable in initiating the process, as it is in accelerating progress after labour has already started.

Explicit rules

The rules which govern the use of oxytocin in this hospital are quite explicit; furthermore, they are rigidly enforced. Extensive practical experience has shown that these rules provide a highly effective series of safeguards:

- A standard concentration of 10 units of oxytocin in 1 litre of dextrose solution is used in all circumstances.
- The total dose of oxytocin received may not exceed 10 units.
- The rate of infusion may not exceed 60 drops per minute. (The drip set conforms with British standard specification, which requires that 15 to 20 drops are equivalent to 1 ml. The maximum dose of oxytocin at 60 drops, therefore, is 40 milliunits/minute.)
- Infusion of 1 litre at the prescribed rate imposes a time limit of 6 hours.

The only variable factor is the rate of infusion; this begins at 10 drops and increases by 10 drops, at intervals of 15 minutes, to a maximum of 60 drops. The rate of infusion attains the maximum level, 60 drops, in the shortest time, 75 minutes, in almost every instance. Evidence of fetal distress is the only absolute bar to this step by step method of progression. See *Graph 19*.

Hypertonic uterine action

The personal nurse – who accompanies everyone in labour – records each contraction as it occurs. The reverse side of the partograph is used for the purpose. The timescale is divided into intervals of 15 minutes. The optimum number of contractions is five. To guard against hypertonus the number of contractions is not permitted to exceed seven in 15 minutes.

Special care is taken to ensure that the mother does not control the drip. In practice, this occurs when the attendant reduces the rate of infusion simply because the mother complains of pain, which is, of course, to be expected. Such indecision is a common manifestation of a low level of confidence in the system, which usually derives from imprecise instructions or lack of trust.

Special equipment

No special equipment is used, either to dispense oxytocin or to monitor its effects. Oxytocin is dispensed from a simple gravity feed, which is regulated by the personal nurse. There is no inherent objection to automation, provided this does not become a mechanical substitute for individual attention. However, it is a mistake to think that a precise dose of oxytocin, in milliunits, offers any material advantage. This is an item of utmost practical importance in centres where special equipment may not be available.

The overall contribution of a personal nurse to a woman in labour extends far beyond supervision of oxytocin in the relatively few cases where this is given, while the answer to the suggestion which is not infrequently made, that it is not feasible to provide personal attention on such a scale, is to remind the reader that this recommendation emanates from a very busy unit.

Causes of confusion

The situation with regard to oxytocin in some centres is indeed difficult to comprehend. There are several consultant obstetricians, each with a fixed preference for a different regimen for which there is no factual basis. Intuitively, it seems, one consultant feels that 2.5 units of oxytocin is best, another 5 units and another 10 units, and to confuse the matter still further, some use all three consecutively in the same case. This bizarre example of therapeutics, where the dose of a drug is altered both in terms of concentration and in rate of administration, can have few counterparts in medicine. Is it any wonder that those called upon to supervise similar cases in adjoining beds, who are prescribed different concentrations of the same drug to treat the same disorder, should feel utterly confused? And when these complexities are compounded by ominous references to possible cephalopelvic disproportion, rupture of uterus and injury to the child, their position becomes virtually untenable. The only sensible course open to a responsible person placed in such an intolerable position would be to reduce the rate of infusion to an ineffectual level, which is not sufficient to dilate the cervix, and to record hypertonic uterine action or fetal distress as the reason for doing so. This is what frequently occurs in practice, thus giving rise to the mistaken impression that oxytocin is sometimes not an effective method of resolving the problem of slow labour. Staff in this hospital are indemnified against cephalopelvic disproportion, rupture of uterus and injury to the child. Care is taken to avoid reference to these subjects altogether in the present context. Criticism is reserved for those who fail to act decisively to restrict the duration of labour.

Water intoxication

The only direct toxic effect of oxytocin is water intoxication. This classical syndrome – which may result in convulsions, coma and even death – is due to an intrinsic antidiuretic effect of oxytocin, which results in reabsorption of salt-free water from renal tubules. As the name implies, water intoxication is related directly to volume of fluid available. The possibility arises when more than 3 litres of salt-free fluid are administered by the intravenous route. This simply cannot occur when the rules, as previously stated, are followed; the fact that the volume of fluid is restricted to 1 litre provides an absolute guarantee against water intoxication. Naturally, careful notice must also be taken of alternative sources of fluid given intravenously, as for example by an anaesthetist in conjunction with epidural block. This can be an important source of additional fluid, especially when epidural block is misused as a cover for prolonged labour; the longer the labour the greater the volume of fluid infused. Oral fluids do not contribute to the problem of water intoxication because these are regulated by the mother, not imposed upon her.

Water intoxication is far more likely to occur when oxytocin is used to induce labour, because all too often induction is allowed to continue for an indefinite period of time, during which an excessive volume of salt-free fluid may be infused without attracting attention.

Neonatal jaundice

An association between oxytocin and neonatal jaundice has attracted some attention. Studies in this hospital have confirmed that there is an increase in the incidence of neonatal jaundice in cases treated with oxytocin, but they have also shown that this increase is confined to cases in which oxytocin is used to induce labour. There is no increase in cases in which oxytocin is used to accelerate labour already started. The overall increase in the incidence of neonatal jaundice associated with oxytocin, therefore, is a reflection of the relative state of immaturity which results from interruption of the course of pregnancy before its natural conclusion; it is not a direct, toxic, effect of oxytocin. This constitutes yet another example of the need to draw a sharp distinction between induction and acceleration of labour.[6]

Trauma

For many years it has been taught that oxytocin increases the risk of trauma to both mother and child, especially where there may be an element of cephalopelvic disproportion. There is no foundation for this proposition, at least in primigravidae. In primigravidae the opposite is true because efficient uterine action reduces the need for traction, which is the real cause of trauma. There was no case of rupture of uterus in more than 50,000 consecutive primigravidae delivered in this hospital during the years under review. There were only two cases of traumatic intracranial haemorrhage in cephalic presentations which were not delivered by forceps; both occurred in exceptional circumstances. The incidence of traumatic intracranial haemorrhage in cephalic presentations, showed a sharp decline after the present policy of prevention of prolonged labour was introduced. The fundamental difference between primigravidae and multigravidae must be noted once again, since oxytocin is a potent cause of rupture of uterus in parous women. The subject of trauma is considered at greater length in Chapter 14. See also *Tables 4 and 5.*

Hypoxia

Hypoxia is a different proposition. Every contraction of the uterus reduces circulation through the placenta, even during the course of normal labour This presents no serious challenge to a fetus who starts labour with a normal placenta, but it can have grave consequences where placental function is already impaired. A fetus with normal placental function is well equipped to withstand the stress of normal labour, unless an accident like prolapse of cord should occur. The fetus who is likely to suffer from hypoxia during the course of normal labour, is the fetus whose placental function was impaired before labour began. To the fetus, the consequences are the same whether the natural action of the uterus is sufficient to dilate the cervix, or inefficient uterine action is corrected with oxytocin. Since the purpose of oxytocin is to simulate normal uterine action, it follows that circulation through the placenta is reduced; in this sense it is inevitable that oxytocin should contribute to the problem of hypoxia. However, hypoxia is not a direct toxic effect of oxytocin; it is a by-product of efficient uterine action.

Summary

Oxytocin is an extraordinarily effective therapeutic agent for the correction of slow labour, but explicit instructions are necessary to ensure that it is properly used. Oxytocin should be restricted to primigravidae, while malpresentations, hydrocephalus and twins should be excluded. Dosage should not exceed 10 units, volume 1 litre or rate 60 drops per minute. There should be a time limit of 6 hours. Subject to these specifications, fetal hypoxia is the only problem. Hence, oxytocin should never be used when there is evidence of impaired placental function or fetal distress. Water intoxication should not occur. Lack of special equipment is not an acceptable excuse for inept management.

10: Normal and Abnormal Labour (Dystocia)

It may seem strange that the basic parameters of normal labour, to which all who are concerned with management should consciously aspire, are seldom, if ever, clearly defined. Although the final result is unlikely to gain universal acceptance, in every minute detail, this can be an immensely rewarding exercise. An agreed definition of normal labour should be posted in a prominent position in every delivery unit – and classroom – to serve as a clear statement of common purpose. The subject should be considered in broad outline, with controversial items best avoided.

In this hospital, labour is classified as normal when a baby is born through the natural passage, by the efforts of the mother, within a reasonable timespan, provided no harm befalls either party as a result of their experience. Twelve hours is regarded as a reasonable timespan.

Conversely, labour is classified as abnormal when delivery is by caesarean section, or through the natural passage by the efforts of the doctor, when duration exceeds 12 hours, or when some harmful effect befalls either party.

Induction of labour is designated abnormal, as are all operative deliveries. This is not to say that induction, caesarean section and low forceps, or ventouse, are not practised, but rather practised with discretion, and always as the lesser of two evils. Kielland's forceps, however, are not used.

Although at first sight these definitions may appear somewhat unrealistic to those accustomed to think of childbirth in terms of technical procedures, developments in this hospital over the past 25 years have shown that this viewpoint is perfectly tenable.

Abnormal labour, or dystocia, has three possible causes: inefficient uterine action, occipitoposterior position, and cephalopelvic disproportion. These correspond with faults in the passage, in the passenger, and in the forces. Significantly, the order of priority is reversed. Attention is again directed to the fact that the term cephalopelvic disproportion, as used throughout this manual, refers only to primigravidae and, moreover, that malpresentations and malformation are not included under this heading. Malpresentations and malformation are the subject of a separate chapter; these complications may give rise to obstructed labour, which constitutes an entirely different clinical syndrome from disproportion.

There is bound to be a subjective element involved in the differential diagnosis between the three possible causes of abnormal labour in individual cases. Occipitoposterior position is the exception, because in a negative sense, at least, it can be excluded at pelvic examination. Therefore, the main problem lies between inefficient uterine action and cephalopelvic disproportion. In practice, the differential diagnosis between these two causes of abnormal labour continues to be based largely on personal preference. Local custom frequently determines which cases of abnormal labour, or dystocia, are attributed to cephalopelvic disproportion, while X-ray pelvimetries are used to bolster opinions which are largely preconceived. This dubious method of procedure is still very evident in the wide variation in the reported incidence of cephalopelvic disproportion in maternity hospitals which are located in the same geographical region and which appear similar in all other respects. The reported incidence of cephalopelvic disproportion is merely a statement of the number of caesarean sections included under that heading, on an arbitrary basis. This is an implausible method of estimating the true prevalence of a disease, and obviously one on which no reliance can be placed.

Traditionally, cephalopelvic disproportion has been taught, to medical students and pupil midwives, as the most important feature of abnormal labour. This, seemingly, arose out of genuine concern that serious harm might befall both mother and child should the condition be overlooked. As previously stated, this is a fundamental mistake, one for which there is absolutely no clinical support. There can be little doubt that the error arose because cephalopelvic disproportion, in primigravidae, and obstructed labour, in multigravidae, were not recognised as distinct entities, with different causes, different treatment and different results. Even more important in this context was failure to recognise that the primigravid uterus is virtually immune to rupture, whereas the multigravid uterus is rupture prone.

Probably the most significant outcome of active management of labour is that effective uterine action is assured in virtually every case admitted to this hospital, with the result that the problem of cephalopelvic disproportion has been isolated for the first time. Now the differential diagnosis between inefficient uterine action, cephalopelvic disproportion and occipitoposterior position, can be made by a simple process of exclusion. Given a cervix which dilates progressively, and an occiput which is not posterior, a diagnosis of cephalopelvic disproportion can confidently be made.

The causes of abnormal labour, or dystocia, are discussed in Chapters 11, 12 and 13; these should be read in conjunction with this chapter.

Summary

Far too much time and attention is devoted to consideration of individual elements of abnormal labour and how to surmount resultant problems by surgical means, without first defining the basic norms to which all should aspire.

11: Inefficient Uterine Action

Inefficient uterine action is far and away the most common complication of labour in primigravidae. This is certainly not so in multigravidae. A diagnosis of inefficient uterine action in a multigravida should always be viewed with gravest suspicion, because the parous uterus is a highly efficient organ with much less resistance to overcome. Slow progress in a multigravida may well be an expression of obstruction, and obstructed labour in a parous woman is much the commonest cause of rupture of uterus. Essential differences between primigravid and multigravid labour need constant reiteration. The present chapter, on inefficient uterine action, refers to primigravidae only; the contents should be applied to multigravidae with extreme caution.

Definitions

The sole function of the uterus during the first stage of labour, is to cause the cervix to dilate. During the second stage of labour, the sole function of the uterus is to cause the head to descend to the level of the pelvic floor. These disparate functions must not be confused. Pressure on the pelvic floor activates the reflex action of voluntary muscles, which in turn cause the baby to be born. The efficiency of the uterus during labour can be gauged only by its ability to complete these specific functions, each within a reasonable timescale. In other words, the efficiency of the uterus can be measured only in terms of results achieved. These results correlate equally poorly with the subjective element of pain, as felt by the mother, and with the objective strength of contractions, as assessed by her attendant. The success or failure of treatment of inefficient uterine action must not be evaluated in this manner.

Acceptance of oxytocin

Although the means, in the form of oxytocin, have long been available, a systematic approach to treatment of inefficient uterine action has been slow to emerge. The reasons for this delay seem to have been as follows:

- As the first step towards a solution of a problem is accurate definition, failure to submit the syndrome of abnormal labour, or dystocia, to detailed analysis rendered a solution virtually impossible.
- Inefficient uterine action, which is far the most common cause of abnormal labour, was itself complicated by being subdivided into two distinct types: hypotonic and hypertonic inertia. This subdivision was coupled with the warning that although stimulation with oxytocin could be beneficial to the former, it could be detrimental to the latter. There is no basis for this assertion: in clinical practice inefficient uterine action is a single entity, and it is uniformly responsive to stimulation with oxy-

tocin.

• Treatment of inefficient uterine action was further inhibited by the proposition, which amounted almost to an article of faith, that stimulation of the uterus in circumstances in which there was even the faintest possibility of cephalopelvic disproportion, could result in serious injury to both mother and child. As cephalopelvic disproportion can never, strictly speaking, be excluded wholly until labour has come to a successful conclusion, this caveat ensured that oxytocin could not be used to proper effect for fear of dire consequences. Because labour could not be brought to a successful conclusion without efficient uterine action, this gave rise to a classical example of a chicken and egg situation. The result was therapeutic paralysis.

Clinical types

Typically, inefficient uterine action presents as slow dilatation of cervix which continues from the very onset of labour. This persistent pattern of slow dilatation should lead to early diagnosis and prompt treatment, long before dehydration, ketosis, or other evidence of physical and mental exhaustion can make their appearance. Moreover, the cervix of a woman in labour is so predictably responsive to stimulation with oxytocin that, whenever the rate of dilatation does not accelerate sharply, the initial diagnosis of labour is almost certainly wrong. Where little attention is paid to diagnosis of labour such cases are commonplace; they may even create an impression that oxytocin is not a reliable method of treatment. Alternatively, this false impression may derive from the popular confusion between acceleration and induction, where there is no clear indication as to when labour begins. It is of the utmost importance to appreciate that slow dilatation of cervix, as a primary phenomenon, is not at all suggestive of cephalopelvic disproportion.

Much less frequently, inefficient uterine action may develop as a secondary phenomenon, in which case it presents as arrest in dilatation of cervix late in the first stage of labour, after there has been a normal beginning. Secondary arrest in dilatation of cervix is indeed suggestive of cephalopelvic disproportion, but because inefficient uterine action is still a more likely cause, individuals should be treated with oxytocin for a limited period of time before resort is made to caesarean section.

Finally, inefficient uterine action may not develop until the second stage of labour, in which case it presents as failure of the head to descend, after full dilatation has been achieved. The clinical situation is identical with the previous paragraph; hence, oxytocin should be given for a limited period of time before resort is made to caesarean section. Forcible vaginal delivery with forceps should certainly not be undertaken at this juncture, simply because the cervix has reached full dilatation. See *Graphs 13, 14, 15, 16.*

Summary

The outstanding lesson that we have learned about labour in recent years is that efficient uterine action represents the key to normality. Furthermore, efficient uterine action can safely be assured in almost every case, through judicious use of oxytocin. There is one overriding qualification: a clear distinction must be maintained between primigravidae and multigravidae at all times. The assurance of efficient uterine action to every primigravida has had the effect of isolating the problem of cephalopelvic disproportion, as a separate clinical entity, for the first time. The result has been a radical change in the whole approach to the conduct of labour in this hospital.

12: Cephalopelvic Disproportion

The concept of cephalopelvic disproportion has coloured attitudes to childbirth for a very long time.[7] The main reason for this is that cephalopelvic disproportion is coupled, in the collective subconscious of obstetricians, with the threat of rupture of the uterus and injury to the child. Hence it may come as no little surprise to learn that in the whole of recorded clinical experience there is no factual basis for either contention. Of course, this is to presume that the term 'cephalopelvic disproportion' is used correctly to refer to primigravidae only, and not extended, incorrectly, to include multigravidae. Rupture of uterus is a calamity which befalls parous women with obstructed labour, usually caused by malpresentations; it does not affect primigravidae with cephalopelvic disproportion. Moreover, injury to a firstborn child is associated almost exclusively with instrumental delivery. The subject of trauma is discussed at greater length in Chapter 14.

There may have been good reason for the widespread concern about cephalopelvic disproportion when rickets was a common disease, but this situation no longer exists. In retrospect, it now seems to have been an unfortunate coincidence that X-ray pelvimetry was perfected at the same time as the social conditions that gave rise to rickets were eradicated more than a generation ago. This has served to perpetuate a preoccupation with a condition which is hardly ever seen nowadays. At that time, X-ray pelvimetry seemed to provide an objective scientific basis for the study of cephalopelvic disproportion, because it reduced the issue to a simple question of shape and size. These features could be accurately portrayed. A diagnosis of contracted pelvis and, by inference, cephalopelvic disproportion, was compared with an orthopaedic fracture: a straightforward combination of modern equipment and technical expertise. It seemed all too reasonable to assume that accurate measurements of her pelvis could only be helpful to a woman facing childbirth for the first time, just as it would have seemed perverse to suggest that such measurements could, in the event, become a liability. But this has proved in practice to be the case.

The standard procedure in those days was to combine digital assessment of pelvis with a head fitting test, in the case of every primigravida in whom the head had not engaged at, say, 38 weeks. This was combined with X-ray pelvimetry. Then, a formal decision was taken between delivery by elective caesarean section and 'trial of labour'. Frequently this crucial decision, which could have permanent repercussions on a woman's lifestyle, was made, albeit indirectly, by a radiologist who had never even seen the patient. The entire birth process was dominated by architectural nuances.

A 'trial' of labour was carefully documented in advance. Antenatal notes included predictions which were frequently pessimistic and always cautionary in tone. Nowhere was it appreciated that a 'trial of labour' might fail simply because the outcome was prejudiced beforehand, or because an intolerable burden of responsibility was placed on midwives and junior doctors by these reservations so freely expressed by their senior colleagues. There was an absolute bar on the use of oxytocin, because it was taken for granted that stimulation of the uterus in the presence of suspected cephalopelvic disproportion could easily result in serious damage to mother or child. Moreover, whenever the uterus did not function effectively to dilate the cervix, this was seen as a protective mechanism which served only to confirm the original suspicion. Finally, a diagnosis of cephalopelvic disproportion once made was permanent in its effect, so that later children were delivered by elective caesarean section without further consideration. This method of procedure had important long-term implications for the woman and her family, which attracted surprisingly little attention.

On an historical note, it was in this hospital that the operation of symphisiotomy was revived in the 1940s, to offset the commitment to repeat caesarean sections in young mothers with a diagnosis of cephalopelvic disproportion. This practice continued for more than 20 years until active management of labour was introduced in the 1960s. This development ensured efficient uterine action for every nulliparous woman in labour. Soon it became apparent that most women previously treated by symphisiotomy, or caesarean section, after failed 'trial of labour' suffered not from cephalopelvic disproportion, but from inefficient uterine action. Within a few years the recorded incidence of cephalopelvic disproportion had fallen to a small fraction of the previous level. Meanwhile, however, the operation had been transported to other centres, mainly in Africa, where it is still widely practised.

Definition

Cephalopelvic disproportion is a term used only in the context of first-time mothers with normal, vertex, presentations. This restricted use of the term is considered a matter of fundamental importance to the elucidation of the problem. The term cephalopelvic disproportion is, advisedly, not used in the context of later births, nor does it include malpresentations, or certain malformations, whatever the mother's parity. Obstructed labour is a term used to describe a completely different clinical entity which directly involves the fetus: such as brow or shoulder presentation, and hydrocephalus. Here the capacity of the pelvis is not the central issue. Obstructed labour, in a multigravida, is a much more dangerous proposition than cephalopelvic disproportion, in a primigravida, because it is all too likely to lead to serious trauma. Rupture of uterus becomes almost inevitable should the obstruction escape notice and oxytocin be infused to stimulate the parous organ, which is efficient by nature. The mistaken belief that a similar fate might befall a primigravida with cephalopelvic disproportion, or indeed obstruction, stems from the general failure to draw a clear distinction between mothers on grounds of parity.

Diagnosis

No consideration whatever is given to the possibility of cephalopelvic disproportion in the course of routine antenatal care at this hospital. All reference to the subject is consciously excluded. No mention is made in case notes, in the firm belief that this can only have an adverse influence on the eventual outcome. The pelvis is not assessed by clinical means, nor is X-ray pelvimetry ever practised. The result is that elective caesarean section is almost never performed for this indication and, in particular, the term 'trial of labour' is studiously avoided at all times.

The possibility of cephalopelvic disproportion is raised for the first time after the course of labour has proved abnormal. Abnormal labour unfolds as the cervix fails to dilate progressively during the first stage, or the head fails to descend during the second stage. Slow progress early in labour, that is as a primary event, is interpreted invariably as an expression of inefficient uterine action, whereas slow progress as a secondary event, that is late in labour, is interpreted sometimes as an expression of cephalopelvic disproportion. Nonetheless, a diagnosis of cephalopelvic disproportion is not seriously entertained until oxytocin has been infused for a reasonable period of time, to eliminate inefficient uterine action which remains the more likely cause even of secondary arrest. A presumptive diagnosis of cephalopelvic disproportion is made when progress remains unsatisfactory under these conditions, provided that the occiput is not posterior. These are the clinical circumstances in which caesarean section for cephalopelvic disproportion is undertaken in this hospital. No attempt is made to anticipate these events, because attempts to anticipate a diagnosis of cephalopelvic disproportion led to much unnecessary surgical intervention in previous years. See *Graph 24*.

Even so, the final conclusion is postponed until the puerperium when, for the purpose of medical audit, every case of dystocia is formally reviewed. A differential diagnosis between inefficient uterine action, cephalopelvic disproportion and occipitoposterior position is made in the light of all the evidence then available. X-ray pelvimetry may be requested at this late stage, mainly, it must be said, for academic purposes. This conclusion, which is officially recorded on the case notes, strongly influences the mode of delivery on the next occasion.

Also for the purpose of medical records, a diagnosis of cephalopelvic disproportion is positively excluded in each case in which labour is classified as normal, because vaginal delivery has been achieved within 12 hours and there has been no significant injury to mother or child. This means that a formal decision, either for or against a diagnosis of cephalopelvic disproportion, is made in every primigravida delivered. The incidence of cephalopelvic disproportion, based on this comprehensive method of selection, has remained stable at 1 in 250 primigravidae, approximately, for the past 25 years. Yet despite this exceptionally low figure, one in every two cases in which a diagnosis of cephalopelvic disproportion was made had a subsequent vaginal delivery in this hospital. Cephalopelvic disproportion, therefore, is clearly not a common disorder where rigorous standards of diagnosis are applied.

Pelvic deformity

Pelvic deformity is considered to be a separate disorder. Less than 1 in 1,000 women is affected. Almost invariably, the deformity is caused either by a limp in childhood or a crush injury in adult life. Diagnosis presents no problem as individuals declare themselves, either by their gait or by their history of a road traffic accident. These are virtually the only cases delivered by elective caesarean section for reasons of pelvic architecture in this hospital.

Change in practice

Over recent decades no single aspect of obstetric practice in this hospital has undergone such radical change as cephalopelvic disproportion. The change has come about as a result of a combination of factors, chief amongst which are: insistence on precise use of terms, realisation that uterine action is the key to normal birth, and conclusive evidence that oxytocin can be used safely in nulliparous women. Now, it is abundantly clear that all efforts to anticipate a diagnosis of cephalopelvic disproportion are not only misguided, they result in a rate of intervention grossly in excess of the true prevalence of the disease. This represents a classical example of a clinical situation where application of the generally laudable principle of prevention becomes counterproductive in its effects. Hence the term 'trial of labour' has been deleted from our vocabulary, while antenatal pelvimetry is no longer practised. Not even short stature is regarded any longer with suspicion, since small mothers give birth to small babies. This observation seems to have global application, as, for example, in Asia and Africa where western observers tend to place undue emphasis on short stature, without directing equal attention to low birth weight.

Summary

The term cephalopelvic disproportion applies only to primigravidae. Malpresentations and hydrocephalus are specifically excluded from consideration under this heading. The clinical approach to the subject is entirely pragmatic; a prospective diagnosis is never entertained. The possibility is first mooted when labour ceases to progress, but a diagnosis of cephalopelvic disproportion is not addressed seriously until efficient uterine action has been assured for a reasonable period of time. This requires oxytocin, which can be given in the sure knowledge that it does not cause rupture of the primigravid uterus or trauma to the child. Therefore, whereas others may say, 'do not use oxytocin unless cephalopelvic disproportion has been excluded', we say, 'cephalopelvic disproportion cannot be excluded unless oxytocin is used'. A definitive diagnosis is postponed until some days after delivery, when all of the relevant information is available for review.

13: Occipitoposterior Position

Persistent occipitoposterior position is the third, and only other possible cause of abnormal labour, or dystocia. The clinical problems posed are very similar to cephalopelvic disproportion. However, there is one important difference: it is quite a simple matter to determine the position of the occiput by pelvic examination. Diagnosis, in this limited sense, is a straightforward procedure.[8]

Management

In this hospital the same pragmatic approach is adopted to occipitoposterior position as to cephalopelvic disproportion. No attention is paid to position of occiput during the closing weeks of pregnancy, and to avoid giving rise to the impression that position may have an adverse effect on the subsequent course of labour, no record is kept at antenatal clinics. As with cephalopelvic disproportion, experience has shown that the greater the emphasis, the more likely it is that difficulties will follow. The anxious doctor creates his own problems under both these headings.

The clinical significance of posterior position does not come into question until the course of labour has already proved abnormal. This becomes evident when the cervix ceases to dilate during the first stage, or the head fails to descend during the second stage. Slow progress as a primary event, that is early in labour, is always interpreted as an expression of inefficient uterine action, whereas slow progress as a secondary event, that is late in labour, is sometimes interpreted as an expression of cephalopelvic disproportion and sometimes of occipitoposterior position. Even at this late juncture inefficient uterine action is still the most likely cause. Secondary arrest of progress which does not respond to stimulation with oxytocin, given for a reasonable period of time, is attributed to malposition when the occiput is posterior and to cephalopelvic disproportion otherwise. Caesarean section is performed in either event, unless the cervix is fully dilated.

In clinical practice, the most dangerous aspect of persistent posterior position emerges during the second stage of labour, when the temptation to opt for vaginal delivery seems almost irresistible. There are still too many obstetricians who equate full dilatation with the point of no return in labour, when vaginal delivery becomes a challenge to manual dexterity. This attitude leads to forcible rotation and extraction, the manoeuvre which, arguably, carries the greatest risk of trauma to both mother and child in contemporary obstetrics. In this hospital, a case of occipitoposterior position that persists for more than one hour into the second stage of labour is delivered by caesarean section without regard to the fact that the cervix is fully dilated, unless the head is on the pelvic floor and manual rotation can be performed easily or vaginal delivery be effected face to pubis. Forceps are not used to rotate, nor is the head ever displaced upwards for this purpose.

Transverse arrest

The term transverse arrest is widely misconstrued. The normal position of the occiput is in the transverse diameter of the pelvis until the head reaches the level of the ischial spines, which mark the junction between the midstrait and the outlet of the bony structure. The ischial spines also mark the level of transition between phase one and phase two of the second stage of labour, described in Chapter 7, because they provide the attachments of the levator ani muscles which form the floor of the birth canal. At this level the reflex action of voluntary muscles is activated and forward rotation of occiput normally occurs. Rotation is effected by the combined action of uterine and voluntary muscles, and when it fails to occur it is because this composite force is not equal to the task. Hence, arrest in the transverse diameter of the pelvis is not, as the term may seem to imply, the result of physical obstruction but rather the expression of inadequate driving force. Transverse arrest is not the cause of delay: it is the result.

Treatment of transverse arrest, therefore, is simply treatment of delay in second stage. In the case of midtransverse arrest, so-called because the head remains above the level of the ischial spines, oxytocin is infused to improve the action of the uterus and thus propel the head downwards to the level at which rotation naturally occurs. In the case of deep transverse arrest, so-called because the head is already at the level of the ischial spines, manual rotation and routine forceps extraction is permissible. No attempt is made to rotate, and subsequently extract, a head arrested in the midstrait of the pelvis; caesarean section is performed whenever the need for delivery arises in such circumstances.

The widespread misunderstanding which exists in respect of the significance of transverse arrest is reflected in the exaggerated attention paid to minor variations in shape and size of pelvis in centres where antenatal pelvimetry is still common practice. There is an unwarranted assumption that prominent ischial spines may cause deep transverse arrest, with the result that forecasts are made of likely trouble at the pelvic outlet long before labour begins. This is a characteristic feature of the mechanical approach to childbirth, where shape and size of pelvis, rather than functional efficiency of uterus, are the main focus of attention.

Results

Position of occiput is recorded as having an adverse effect on outcome in 1 in every 250 primigravidae delivered in this hospital. By mere coincidence, this is the same figure quoted for cephalopelvic disproportion in Chapter 12. In effect, this means that approximately 8 in every 1,000 primigravidae – less than 1% – do not achieve the goal of safe vaginal delivery within a reasonable period of time, as a consequence of one or other condition. The differential diagnosis is based almost entirely on the position of occiput at the point of delivery and is made, therefore, in retrospect. Although, inevitably, there is some degree of overlap between the two conditions, this does not affect management.

Summary

There is a very close similarity between persistent occipitoposterior position and cephalopelvic disproportion in clinical practice. Special care must be taken not to create problems under either heading by making gratuitous predictions on the eventual outcome of labour. As with cephalopelvic disproportion, forecasts in this direction have a strong tendency to self fulfilment. Posterior position should not be cited as the cause of abnormal labour unless inefficient uterine action has been positively excluded, if necessary with oxytocin. Although posterior position may be associated with slow progress late in the first stage of labour, the main danger arises early in the second stage when there is a strong temptation to attempt vaginal delivery in unfavourable circumstances, before the head has descended to a suitable level.

The term transverse arrest should be discarded; it is a misnomer based on lack of understanding of the natural process of descent and rotation during the course of normal labour.

14: Trauma

Trauma in obstetrics should be considered as a single proposition, because the circumstances which give rise to trauma in the mother are the same as those which give rise to trauma in the child. These arise late in labour and are almost invariably associated with operative intervention at the point of delivery. Breech presentation is the obvious exception: trauma in breech presentation is confined to the fetus and is inherent in the mode of birth.

Injury to mother

Rupture of uterus is the classical example of serious trauma to the mother. This catastrophe is not likely to escape notice because it results in massive blood transfusion, hysterectomy and even death. The first reported case in the medical literature of rupture of uterus in a primigravida, which was not associated with manipulation, occurred in a woman who was treated with oxytocin under cover of epidural anaesthesia, in the course of labour which was allowed to continue for more than 50 hours[9]. The interest in this particular case is that it was reported for the express purpose of refuting our statement that the primigravid uterus is virtually immune to rupture, except by manipulation. It could have been presented much more suitably as a bizarre exception to prove that general rule. There was, of course, no case of ruptured uterus in more than 50,000 consecutive primigravidae delivered in this hospital during the period under review, despite extensive use of oxytocin to accelerate progress in some 20,000 primigravidae, in both first and second stages of labour. See *Table 4*.

Laceration of cervix, rupture of vault, and spiral tears of vagina are somewhat less dramatic manifestations of serious trauma to the mother which also may entail profuse haemorrhage, blood transfusion and extensive surgical repair. Although not so easy to quantify accurately in numerical terms, these injuries are likewise associated almost exclusively with assisted vaginal delivery, especially where forceps are used for the purpose of rotation in phase one of the second stage of labour.

Injury to child

Rupture of tentorium cerebelli is the classic example of serious trauma to the child. This lesion, which results in subdural haemorrhage, can be demonstrated at autopsy and affords conclusive evidence of cause of death. Rupture of tentorium has a special association with breech presentation; this is one of the main reasons why all malpresentations are excluded from consideration in this manual. Equally important, but not so well known, is the fact that virtually every case of injury to the tentorium that is not associated with breech presentation, is associated with instrumental vaginal delivery.

There were 44 fatal cases of traumatic intracranial haemorrhage in firstborn infants delivered in this hospital during the period 1963–1979 inclusive: 27 cephalic and 17 breech presentations. All 27 cephalic presentations were delivered with forceps. There was no case of traumatic intracranial haemorrhage other than in breech or forceps delivery. This unequivocal statement is based firmly on the comprehensive post-mortem coverage achieved during those years.[10]

The close correlation between trauma in the mother and trauma in the child is clearly illustrated by the 27 cases of traumatic intracranial haemorrhage in cephalic presentations described in the previous paragraph. The outcome in the 27 mothers was as follows: one death, eight blood transfusions for traumatic haemorrhage, one persistent foot-drop, and three retained in hospital for more than 2 weeks. This represents a total of 13 individuals, or almost 50%. Inexperience was not a factor in these cases: the forceps were applied by a consultant in 10, senior registrar in 14 and junior medical officer in three cases only. A clear association between trauma and duration is evident from the fact that labour was prolonged, more than 12 hours, in no less than 16 of the 27 cases.[10]

Prevention of trauma

A sharp decline in the incidence of trauma occurred after the decision was taken to limit the duration of labour to 12 hours in this hospital. Meanwhile, although the manoeuvre of rotation with forceps was completely discarded, no increase in the number of caesarean sections followed. The probable explanation is that more babies are born by propulsion and fewer by traction, especially combined with rotation.

An apparent anomaly in contemporary attitudes to the fetus during labour is the contrast which sometimes exists between a high level of attention paid to hypoxia, and an almost casual approach to trauma. A fetus supervised with meticulous care through pregnancy and first stage of labour is subjected to a degree of trauma at the point of delivery which would not be considered tolerable under any circumstances a few hours later. Forcible extraction is undertaken, sometimes for no better reason than that the cervix is fully dilated for a specified period. At other times trauma is inflicted in the course of a frantic effort to rescue the fetus from a condition of distress based on slender evidence. The doctor, understandably anxious to save the fetus from hypoxia, exposes it to trauma, and introduces the risk of serious injury to the mother in the process. Perinatal death in such circumstances is almost sure to be attributed to hypoxia unless an autopsy is performed, and even so it is often wrongly assumed that intracranial haemorrhage was the cause of fetal distress rather than the result of treatment. The sequence of errors is complete when rupture of tentorium, which leads to intracranial haemorrhage, is attributed to cephalopelvic disproportion. Cephalopelvic disproportion is certainly not a significant factor in the aetiology of trauma in obstetrics.

Fourteen of the 27 mothers referred to above returned to this hospital for their second birth: 13 had a spontaneous delivery of a healthy infant, which, incidentally, weighed more than the first in 11 instances. Moreover, six of the 27 first-born infants were preterm, thus confirming the general belief that preterm infants are more vulnerable to trauma. However, it is worthy of special notice that these were the only preterm infants who died from intracranial haemorrhage in this hospital over this entire period of 17 years; all were delivered with forceps. This points to the inevitable conclusion that it was the forceps, not the immaturity, which was the decisive factor. Consequently, the practice of routine delivery of preterm infants with forceps is not to be recommended as a prophylactic measure against trauma.[10]

Summary

Breech presentation apart, trauma in obstetrics is associated to an over-whelming degree with instrumental delivery. Trauma, therefore, is much more common in primigravidae. The use of oxytocin to ensure efficient uterine action reduces the need for traction, because it supports the natural process of propulsion which enables primigravidae to deliver themselves. Forceps do not protect the immature head from trauma.

15: Pain

The most characteristic feature of the conventional attitude towards management of labour is the strong emphasis placed on the element of pain and, consequently, on drugs for relief of pain. There are many delivery units which operate from the simple premise that virtually the only, and certainly the most valuable, contribution a midwife or doctor can make to the comfort of a woman in labour, is to ensure that she receives analgesic agents in adequate amounts. This passive attitude to management has led to widespread abuse of drugs; the results are far from impressive, even in the short-term sense of immediate consumer satisfaction. That there is a physical element in the discomfort of labour is not open to question, but it is equally true that the nature of the pain of labour is patently different from the pain associated with surgical operations, or other form of injury for which similar remedies are prescribed.[11]

First stage

Pain in the first stage of labour is intermittent, lasts not longer than one minute, then ceases completely. Approximately five such pains recur at regular intervals in each period of 15 minutes; this amounts to a total of 100 pains during the course of a first labour of average duration. Pains occur somewhat less frequently at the beginning, and more frequently at the end. The type of pain is a cramp, comparable with primary spasmodic dysmenorrhoea, with which almost every woman is familiar.

The nature of discomfort during the first stage is quite different from the nature of discomfort during the second stage. An important component of discomfort during the first stage of labour derives from a mounting sense of frustration which a woman often endures because she feels herself to be a helpless victim of powerful natural forces, over which she can exercise little influence. Swept along on a tide of events, the purpose of which she may not fully comprehend, she tends to lose self control. This is especially so when progress is slow and no one can say when her ordeal is likely to come to an end. Meanwhile, staff come and go at regular intervals of eight hours, when for her the problem seems to begin all over again. For these special reasons, and because of its comparatively long duration, the problem of pain in labour is essentially a problem of the first stage: the tedious hours while the cervix dilates. In this respect, yet again, a first labour is unique. Acceleration with oxytocin, therefore, is often more constructive than analgesia in relief of this discomfort. A dramatic improvement in the outlook of a woman in labour can be expected when the impasse which results from inefficient uterine action is broken and progress is restored – and this despite the fact that contractions are now much stronger.

Second stage

Although the physical element of discomfort is much more in evidence during the second stage of labour, a woman is generally better able to cope because she is actively engaged. Now she senses that the end is near and, moreover, that it can be hastened by her own efforts. She can regain a measure of control of the situation as the tremendous physical exertion required in pushing, distracts her attention from the uterine contractions. A priori, it must be assumed that almost every woman would wish to give birth to her own child. Few women, irrespective of appearances at the critical time, would wish the doctor to act as surrogate mother in this respect.

Reaction to pain

Women seem to react to the pain of labour in an instinctive manner; initially startled, then tense, then restive and finally limp, when with eyes tightly closed they tend to withdraw completely from contact with their surroundings. The intensity of the reaction grows with successive pains until it extends to fill the interval between contractions so that there is no longer any period of relaxation. This scenario, where a woman continues to react long after a contraction has passed, should not be allowed to develop further because contact once lost is seldom possible to restore. Loss of contact with a woman in labour is usually a product of poor management, to which analgesic drugs are not the appropriate answer.

Surely the most impressive feature of pain in labour, however, is the extraordinary variation in the type of reaction of different individuals to what is, in effect, the same stimulus. Although objective measurements may indicate uterine contractions of similar frequency, similar strength and similar duration, the very wide range in response of different individuals affords clear evidence of the paramount importance of the subjective element in the pain of labour. Emotional stability is invariably put to the test at times of stress, and there is no stress in the lifetime of an average person, man or woman, to compare with the birth of a first child. Hence the whole spectrum of human behaviour is revealed in a busy delivery unit in the course of a single day. To concentrate attention on the physical element of the pain of labour, to the virtual exclusion of the nature of the subjective response, is comparable to concentrating on the virulence of the organism in a case of infection, without due regard to the resistance of the host. In general terms, much more can be achieved through action taken to raise the level of resistance to stress than can be achieved by the use of analgesic drugs. This too is the humane way, because it leaves a woman in full control of her faculties, enhances her sense of dignity and permits her to give birth to her own child. In an ideal world, there would be no need for drugs at this critical juncture in one's life. Although this happy state may appear quite unrealistic to many, it should be noted that almost 50% of primigravidae delivered in this hospital receive no medication. In this context, the signal importance attached to duration of exposure, and to continuous personal support through labour, are discussed in Chapters 4 and 19.

In this hospital, no analgesia is given until a firm diagnosis of labour is made and, therefore, a woman is committed to delivery. This is an absolute imperative and evasions are not tolerated under the guise of ambivalent terms such as false or latent labour. The use of analgesic drugs on speculative grounds, to see what may subsequently transpire, is utterly condemned. A drug given in these circumstances gravely confuses the clinical picture for mother and staff alike. The effect is to commit the woman to delivery, even though she may not be in labour. Eventually this can result in an unnecessary caesarean section. Whosoever administers the first drug in a delivery unit assumes a grave responsibility and should, therefore, be made acutely conscious of the possible adverse consequences of their untimely action.

Preparation

A woman's attitude to childbirth reflects many and varied influences to which she has been exposed since early childhood. No short-term course of lectures is likely to result in a radical change of outlook so deeply entrenched. Nevertheless, it would be difficult to exaggerate the importance attached to antenatal education in the alleviation of pain in labour in this hospital. The overall purpose is to convince the expectant mother that she has nothing to fear, and that she is perfectly capable of giving birth to her own child. This is subject always to two firm commitments: that duration of labour is strictly limited and that personal attention is available at all times. Consciously or otherwise, these are the two considerations which weigh most heavily on the minds of ordinary women confronted with the birth of a first child. Consequently, no effort is spared to ensure that every primigravida attends these antenatal classes, on the mutual understanding that the first experience of childbirth is a matter of monumental importance to the future happiness of an entire family.

Summary

Relief of pain in labour is considered under four separate headings: antenatal education, personal attention, limited duration and analgesia. The ability to restrict duration is crucial, because duration of exposure to stress is the dominant element in the problem of pain in labour. Duration has repercussions under each of the other three headings too: education suffers serious loss of credibility when teachers are unable to state duration without the customary evasions; personal attention cannot be provided for everyone unless the timespan is limited; dosage of analgesic drugs corresponds closely with number of hours spent in a labour ward. Individual chapters are devoted to each of these four items.

16: Antenatal Preparation

Although few obstetricians, nowadays, may wish to appear openly hostile to the principle of preparation for childbirth, many continue to pay lip service only to the ideal while taking no interest whatever in the practice. This is yet another characteristic feature of the passive approach to management of labour where, hopefully, everything will come right on the day, and should this prove not to be the case, there are few problems not amenable to treatment with analgesia – provided enough is given and by the proper route – failing which, there is always caesarean section. This can fittingly be described as the 'less one knows the better' school of thought, which stems from lack of direct involvement in labour management.

The almost total neglect of antenatal preparation as a legitimate topic for discussion in academic circles, with the consequent lack of any authoritative guidance on organisation, content or even personnel, is indicative of the state of apathy which exists within the medical establishment regarding this important subject. Meanwhile, obstetric physiotherapists, in particular, are left very much to themselves, suffering greatly as a consequence, both in terms of job satisfaction for the individual and professional status for the group. Direct involvement in management, on the other hand, can only lead to the conclusion that antenatal preparation is an absolutely essential element of quality care in labour.

Purpose

The main purpose of antenatal preparation is, and should always be seen to be, to define a woman's role in labour and to teach her how to fulfil it. There are two distinct, albeit closely related, components: education and training. The educational component should seek to ensure that every expectant mother has a broad understanding of the birth process, while the training component should aim to teach her how to achieve the ultimate prize of spontaneous delivery.

Practice

In this hospital, expectant mothers are encouraged strongly in the belief that they are well able to give birth to their own children. Thus, a spirit of self reliance is consciously nurtured. Two firm assurances are deemed necessary: that continuous, sympathetic and informed support will be forthcoming, and that labour will not be allowed to last too long.

Content

The educational component is based on a clear description of the first and second stages of labour, couched in simple language which a lay person of reasonable intelligence can readily understand: how the first stage is concerned solely with opening of the neck of the womb, a comparatively long and tedious preliminary process over which the mother has virtually no control, and how the second stage is concerned with passage of the infant through the birth canal culminating in the actual birth, a short and somewhat turbulent process which can be brought to a rapid conclusion by the mother's own, not inconsiderable, efforts. A particular point to which great importance is attached, is that everyone should be prepared for the oftimes cataclysmic sensation of sudden pressure on the pelvic floor, which marks the transition between phase one and phase two of the second stage of labour. This is a dramatic event which can have an altogether devastating effect when it occurs without adequate warning.

The concept of graphic representation of labour is explained in some detail, and expectant mothers are shown how this procedure is utilised to record rate of progress and forecast time of delivery. Everyone is given a copy of the official partograph to take away for further study, and all are expected to be familiar with the regimen when admitted eventually in labour. The simple coloured partograph, illustrated in Section II, has proved an invaluable educational instrument in this, lay, context.

The common forms of medical intervention and the reasons are explained: artificial rupture of membranes, oxytocin infusion, low forceps application and episiotomy. A sharp distinction is made between induction of labour and treatment of abnormal uterine action after labour has begun.

Pain is discussed as a subsidiary item. To place pain in its natural sequence, attention is drawn to Braxton Hicks contractions of uterus, which are very noticeable during late pregnancy, and an explanation is given for the close affinity with the contractions of uterus during labour. The effect of anxiety on the threshold for pain is frankly discussed, but care is taken not to make pain appear a central issue lest a serious disservice be done, which could indeed justify the criticism that some antenatal classes are worse than none, because women are left even more apprehensive than before. This is yet another expression of a negative, or passive, attitude towards labour.

The steps taken to supervise the welfare of the fetus are demonstrated: colour of liquor and direct auscultation, as routine, extending to include electronic monitor, scalp electrode and capillary blood sample, in special circumstances.

Three specific items are regarded as of such outstanding practical importance that they are tested in the form of direct question and answer, as follows:

Question: How will you know when to go to hospital in labour?
Answer: When I get painful contractions which resemble period pains, together with a show or persistent leakage of water—or, failing either of these, when the pains come at regular intervals of 10 minutes or less.
Question: How long will you be there before your baby is born?
Answer: Six hours on average, never longer than 12.
Question: Will you ever be left alone?
Answer: Never.

That every woman approaching the birth of her first child should be in possession of these basic facts is considered to be the best simple assessment of the relevance of her preparation.

The training component of antenatal preparation is based on learning how to relax as the uterus contracts, during the first stage, and how to reinforce the natural expulsive forces as the head impacts on the pelvic floor, during the second stage.

Organisation

As in other areas of medical activity, careful planning can make all the difference between success and comparative failure. In this hospital, attention is concentrated on primigravidae, who form a homogenous group of expectant mothers with special problems which they approach largely with an open mind. Almost all series of classes are confined to primigravidae, on the basis of the proposition that if one looks after first time mothers well, the others will look after themselves. Multigravidae are segregated because, as a group, their problems are quite different, while, in addition, they are not infrequently prejudiced by past events. A parous woman who seeks assistance of this nature, especially for the first time, is likely to be motivated by an unfortunate previous episode. This sequence of events can have an unsettling effect on her primigravid sisters, especially when she is anxious to recount her own experience and thus undermine the position of the teacher whenever descriptions given in class do not correspond exactly with her personal memories in every detail. Parous women tend to have closed minds on the subject of labour. They are wont to extrapolate from what is a unique occasion, in terms of individual experience, and they are frequently mistaken in the belief that others placed in a similar situation would necessarily share the same viewpoint; they do not, in a word, appreciate that women differ as much as labours differ. Courses for multigravidae are, therefore, held separately. Indeed, a constant theme stressed in every chapter of this manual is the need to recognise fundamental differences between primigravidae and multigravidae, in everything which relates to labour. Antenatal education, too, must take these differences into account.

In the case of a multigravida the main purpose of the teacher should be to convince her of the truth of the simple maxim: that a first and a subsequent labour are not in any way comparable. As this is primarily an exercise in rehabilitation, it is well to appreciate that uncritical approval of epidural anaesthesia to solve a problem which does not exist in reality, undermines a woman's confidence even further, no matter how grateful she may appear to be.

In this hospital, classes are arranged to correspond with antenatal clinics, so that it is possible to attend both, at the same visit and with the minimum of inconvenience. Attendance is limited to 24 mothers. In total, 13 courses are run concurrently, each morning and afternoon; only two are for multigravidae. Courses begin at 30 weeks, so that the recently acquired knowledge may remain fresh in mind. Discussion is encouraged, but much time is saved by anticipating the questions which are sure to be asked. Six sessions of one hour are devoted to labour. The number of classes is purposely restricted because as classes increase in number so do defaulters. Limiting the number of classes also helps concentrate the attention of both audience and teacher, and thus reduces the tendency to boredom. Three classes are devoted to an understanding of the physical process of childbirth and three classes to the practice of relaxation and propulsion, at the appropriate stages. A documentary film is shown at which husbands are welcome. Finally, there is a conducted tour of the delivery unit. Almost 80% of primigravidae avail of the complete package.

Personnel

To achieve full potential, antenatal education must be conducted under enlightened medical supervision, to ensure that the efforts of teachers are coordinated and that the content is relevant to clinical practice in the particular institution. This is to presume that clinical practice is consistent; otherwise, it is difficult to imagine how teachers can function effectively. Individual teachers should be midwives or physiotherapists who have ongoing practical experience in the delivery unit in question. These two disciplines correspond broadly with the educational and training components previously mentioned. No teacher should be engaged exclusively in this area because this, inevitably, leads to a condition of isolation, which is one of the main factors militating against proper recognition of educational programmes of this nature.

As mutual confidence is the keynote, this requires that teachers appear to know precisely what they are talking about in strictly medical terms, and in relation to actual practice in the particular institution. Naturally, they should also have insight into the anxieties peculiar to a group of women faced with the challenge of a lifetime. Incidentally, teachers should be acutely conscious of the exceptional opportunity afforded them to provide a favourable image of the entire obstetric service to the consumers. Too often teachers and practitioners appear to be almost in direct conflict with each other, because they have developed little or no common ground.

Summary

Antenatal classes have now been available on an organised basis over a considerable period of time without meeting with the general level of acceptance which they so clearly deserve. There are genuine reasons for this comparative failure which need to be examined carefully with a view to placing the service on a more acceptable footing all round. Such a development would be of enormous benefit to everyone concerned with the conduct of labour. The ambivalent nature of medical opinion on the subject seems to derive mainly from the conviction that much of what is taught is irrelevant, if not downright harmful; this is met by the countercharge that there is very little, in the form of consistent medical practice, to be relevant *to*, in most institutions. The worst feature of all is the frequency with which two indispensable arms of the same hospital service seem to operate at virtual loggerheads.

17: Analgesic Drugs

Pethidine, or demoral, is the standard drug for relief of pain in labour, used almost everywhere. Although far from ideal for the purpose, pethidine has been tested on such an extensive scale that it is generally agreed to be about the best drug available, while comparatively safe in reasonable doses. As safety is of paramount importance, particularly in relation to the child, this should preclude the use of new preparations until exhaustive clinical trials have been conducted. It is notable that despite innumerable initial claims to the contrary, no drug has yet emerged to challenge the dominant position of pethidine seriously over many years. The reason is that the ability of a drug to relieve pain is in direct proportion to its potential adverse effects, especially on the respiratory centre of the newborn. Pethidine is the only drug used to relieve pain in labour in this hospital.

Disadvantages of pethidine

Pethidine has many disadvantages which are wholly unpredictable in individual cases. Some women suffer from intractable nausea and vomiting, sufficient to turn childbirth into a miserable experience. Some become profoundly depressed, introspective, and so overwhelmed with self pity that they lapse eventually into a state of stupor, from which they are roused only by contractions, to make aimless protests and demand more and more drugs, until the original situation is compounded and a vicious circle is established. Some become completely disorientated and so confused that they are quite unable to cooperate with their attendants, especially during the second stage of labour, when cooperation is essential if spontaneous delivery is to be achieved. Spontaneous delivery represents an important personal achievement of which mothers should not be deprived lightly; it also provides the best possible insurance against trauma.

In practice, many women in labour are deeply intoxicated; out of bed, they would be unable to stand upright and would certainly be deemed unfit to drive a motor car. Like drunken folk everywhere they are likely to suffer from a hangover: a most undesirable sequel to such a joyous occasion as the birth of a first child. All these adverse effects may follow even a small dose of pethidine given to a person who has had no previous exposure to hard drugs. Unfortunately, the unpleasant side effects of pethidine have become too closely identified with childbirth itself, in the popular perception. Paradoxically, this leads to an even greater demand for drugs.

The most serious adverse effect of pethidine is on the child. Depression of the respiratory centre may delay the establishment of normal breathing in the critical minutes after birth. This can result in permanent brain damage, especially in preterm infants and where adequate facilities for resuscitation are not immediately available. Sophisticated methods of examination reveal subtle changes in behaviour of the new-born after what most obstetricians would regard as homeopathic doses of pethidine. These changes raise the question as to whether pethidine, however small the dose, is ever entirely safe for the child.

A question which needs to be addressed seriously is whether the advantages of pethidine are outweighed by the disadvantages to the extent that the use of pethidine in labour should be discontinued completely. The plain fact of the matter is that it is simply not possible to provide sufficient pethidine to relieve pain in labour effectively without introducing an extraneous element of discomfort and, sometimes, danger. The problem is that there is no more suitable drug available. Relief of pain in labour, therefore, must of necessity entail a genuine compromise between a reasonable degree of analgesia and a reasonable element of iatrogenic discomfort, in the case of the mother, with possible depression of the nervous system, in the case of the child.

A number of drugs have been recommended in combination with pethidine, in the hope that they might enhance the desirable effects or neutralise the undesirable. None has proved successful. As a matter of medical principle, drugs in combination are best avoided; they cross the placenta, may confuse the diagnosis of fetal distress and can cause problems in the newborn which endure for a considerable time: diazepam, which can be detected weeks later, is a classical example.

Naloxone is a special substance; it is a specific opiate antagonist which competes at receptor level and therefore reverses all the effects of pethidine, including the desired analgesic effect, within minutes of injection. Consequently, although its application during labour is clearly limited, it can be invaluable after delivery, particularly in reversing pethidine induced respiratory depression in the newborn. The only drawback seems to be a short half-life which could mean that continuous infusion is required over a protracted period. Naloxone should be instantly available wherever pethidine is used.

Use of pethidine

Pethidine should not be used on a routine basis simply to comply with some obstetric ritual, or to protect staff from possible criticism later. A doctor who appears critical of a midwife because an occasional woman subsequently complains that she has not had sufficient pain relief, encourages this form of mass medication. Doctors are seldom present to witness the particular circumstances and it is all too easy for them to pose as being more humane, after the event. No personal commitment is required for this mode of behaviour. The strongest arguments in favour of large doses of analgesic drugs during labour are advanced mostly by doctors who do not themselves spend much time in a delivery unit. Pethidine, it must be strongly emphasised, often makes labour more unpleasant than it otherwise would have been; moreover, the more pethidine a woman receives, the more disgruntled she often becomes.

Indeed, the woman who complains most vehemently, both during and after the event, is not infrequently herself the victim of a surfeit of drugs.

The practice in this hospital is to await the reaction of every woman to her unique personal experience of labour. Each one is treated as an individual in this respect. Expectant mothers are advised that all methods of pain relief are available, but that prior commitments are not given because this is considered not to serve the best interest of the individual. Expectant mothers are, however, given a firm assurance that the duration of exposure will be strictly limited and that a personal nurse will be present at all times: they are, in other words, encouraged to consider the problem of pain relief in a wider context. The result is that almost one-half of all primigravidae request no analgesic drugs during labour.

First stage

Pethidine is given only with the informed consent of the mother, and during the first stage of labour. The initial dose is 50 mg, which serves as a test dose to assess the individual response. A small dose is preferred because, should a large dose be given and side effects follow, the error cannot so easily be rectified. Adequate relief for the duration of the first stage of labour is provided by a single injection of 50 mg in most cases. A second injection is given half an hour later if the desired effect is not achieved and side effects are not troublesome. The total dose of pethidine does not exceed 100 mg and whenever this proves insufficient an epidural block is introduced. Pethidine in excess of 100 mg tends to cause more discomfort than it relieves. No alternative substance is used, and no combination is permitted. This exercise of strict control over the distribution of analgesic agents fosters a more constructive approach to the overall problem of stress in labour.

Second stage

There is not nearly the same need for analgesia during the second stage of labour, because during contractions mothers are usually preoccupied with the immediate task in hand. This distraction operates as a most effective method of pain relief. The sense of frustration which is so characteristic of the first stage is now replaced by bursts of almost frenzied activity, through which a woman can largely determine her own fate. Properly harnessed, this sense of active participation can alter the whole outlook. There are two exceptions to these general observations: for the duration of phase one, before the head has descended to the level at which the push reflex is activated, no additional analgesia is required because this is simply an extension of the first stage of labour, and late in phase two, as the head crowns, when there is clearly a need for much more effective analgesia.

Inhalation analgesia, in the form of nitrous oxide, which is self-administered, is confined to phase two of the second stage of labour, and is used, therefore, for a relatively short period; prolonged exposure to nitrous oxide may result in hyperventilation with alkalosis and dehydration, apart from a severe hangover. During the hectic moments, as the head crowns, the benefit which accrues from this form of analgesia seems to derive at least as much from the inducement to breathe in and out, rather than push, as from the direct effect of the gas itself.

Forceps extraction is conducted under pudendal block, for two main reasons: first to eliminate the not inconsiderable risk of a general anaesthetic administered to a woman advanced in labour and, second, to restrict the scope for manoeuvre by the operator, with consequent reduction in the likelihood of trauma. There is, in addition, the practical advantage of not requiring the presence of an anaesthetist. Rotation with forceps is not permitted, and for this reason Kielland's forceps are not available in this hospital.

Summary

The ideal drug for pain relief in labour does not exist. Meanwhile, pethidine seems the best available, but it remains open to serious question whether, in balance, pethidine may cause more discomfort than it relieves. A far more critical approach to the whole question of drugs in labour is desirable. No drug whatever should be given before a firm diagnosis of labour has been made and the woman, therefore, is committed to delivery. Pain should not be considered as a separate problem in complete isolation from other relevant aspects of the birth process. Alternative methods of relief – antenatal preparation, personal attention and control of duration – offer much brighter prospects for success.

18: Epidural Anaesthesia

Epidural anaesthesia, as the term implies, affords complete relief of pain in all but a few instances, and has the decided additional advantage that it is not associated with any of the unpleasant side effects of pethidine. The mother retains her mental acuity and the infant is alert at birth. There are few more impressive sights than the resolution of maternal distress which follows a successful epidural block in labour. The answer to the problem of maternal stress in labour might, therefore, appear simple: make epidural anaesthesia available on a comprehensive scale and encourage everyone to avail of the service. However, this would be a gross over simplification of a much more complex problem because, although epidural block is far more effective than pethidine, it is also far more dangerous. No good purpose is served by pretending otherwise. The dangers of epidural block can be considered under two headings: direct effects of a local anaesthetic agent placed in the epidural space, and indirect effects of the anaesthesia on the course of labour.

Direct adverse effects

The main danger of epidural block is accidental entry of the anaesthetic agent into the cerebrospinal fluid. This can lead to profound depression of vital centres, collapse of circulation and even death. There is also the possibility of permanent damage among survivors. The likelihood of a disaster of such magnitude depends largely on the skill and experience of the anaesthetist, but it cannot be excluded entirely because the mechanism is inherent in the procedure itself. The risk of any form of medical intervention in current obstetric practice must be measured against the background of one maternal death for every 10,000 babies born. Two deaths in a series of 10,000 mothers who received an epidural block would represent an increase of 100% in the maternal mortality rate in developed countries. No series of this magnitude has been published, and if it were it would still be less than adequate from a statistical viewpoint. Published series, moreover, are almost always presented by specialist anaesthetists operating under ideal conditions in teaching hospitals. Furthermore they are concerned only with the direct effects of the procedure, which fall within their own competence. Even so, there is a notable reluctance to publish details of maternal catastrophes which occur in association with epidural anaesthesia, and an understandable tendency to attribute these to intercurrent disease such as toxaemia, haemorrhage or ruptured uterus, wherever possible, without sufficient regard to the fact that epidural block can play a critical role in the response of the organism to these conditions. There is a grey area between anaesthetics and obstetrics into which not a few disasters of childbirth fall.

The inevitable loss of mobility associated with epidural block can be a considerable disadvantage to women who otherwise would have elected to remain ambulant during labour, while intractable headache following dural tap, and retention of urine requiring repeated catheterisation, are unpleasant consequences encountered more frequently than is generally appreciated in postnatal wards. In addition, abnormalities of the fetal heart rate resulting from epidural anaesthetic may result in emergency caesarean section.

Indirect adverse effects

The obstetrician must, in addition, be concerned with the indirect effects of epidural block on the course of labour. This is an aspect of the procedure to which far too little attention is paid.

Sometimes epidural block is given too early, before a firm diagnosis of labour is established. The result is that after much confusion, a caesarean section is eventually performed on a woman who is not in labour, because it is well nigh impossible to withdraw the anaesthetic before delivery. Usually the mistake is not recognised, but even so the obstetrician would be understandably slow to admit that a woman has had an unnecessary caesarean section to retrieve a situation caused by a palliative procedure, the implications of which she may not have fully understood. Although the operation is performed to retrieve an iatrogenic situation, the indication for caesarean section is almost sure to be attributed to lack of progress in labour. The effect of this is to transfer the onus to the recipient. Hence, an epidural anaesthetic should never be given until a diagnosis of labour is firmly established and the woman is, therefore, committed to delivery. Effectively, this should preclude epidural anaesthesia before an attempt is made to induce labour.

Sometimes epidural anaesthesia is given too late, when the cervix is close to full dilatation. The result is that the beneficial effects in the first stage are more than offset by the adverse effects in the second stage. The benefits of the procedure are reaped almost entirely during the first stage of labour, while the price is paid largely during the second stage. This price is manifest in the form of a sharp increase in the number of forceps extractions, with the associated risk of trauma. The problem of the late epidural is most likely to arise in the case of a parous woman to whom a prior commitment has been made and who in the event, expects the commitment to be honoured, come what may. This is especially likely when an element of subtle persuasion has been used to influence the woman to the viewpoint that epidural anaesthesia is necessary to make childbirth a tolerable experience.

Sometimes epidural anaesthesia is used as a palliative procedure, when labour is prolonged, as if duration of itself were not important, provided the mother suffers no pain. This approach to the subject of pain illustrates the fundamental difference between the philosophies which underlie active and passive management of labour. Active management of labour is based on the proposition that the risks increase proportionately with the duration of labour, whether or not a woman suffers pain. Indeed, total relief of pain can create a sense of false security when labour is prolonged. Rupture of uterus is the ultimate expression of trauma in the mother, and epidural anaesthesia has emerged as an important factor in the aetiology of this calamity in recent years. Rupture of uterus is virtually confined to multigravidae and it is very significant that the first case of rupture of uterus attributed to oxytocin in a primigravida occurred under cover of epidural anaesthesia after more than 50 hours in labour, as recounted in Chapter 14. This was a classic example of the misuse of epidural anaesthesia to permit the duration of labour to be extended for a dangerous length of time. Ironically, the declared purpose of the publication was to show that it is possible to rupture a primigravid uterus with oxytocin. The strongest possible recommendation is that epidural anaesthesia should not be used as a substitute for corrective action in prolonged labour.

Epidural anaesthesia usually results in a sharp increase in the number of forceps deliveries. About 10% of primigravidae are delivered with forceps in this hospital, compared with as many as 70% in some centres where epidural anaesthesia is freely used. Traumatic intracranial haemorrhage is the ultimate expression of trauma in the child. Apart from breech presentation, this is associated almost invariably with forceps extraction. The risk is greatest when the head is transverse and rotation is required, but it cannot be emphasised sufficiently that trauma in cephalic presentation is inflicted with instruments; it is not a problem in spontaneous delivery. Epidural anaesthesia, therefore, has an important bearing on trauma to the child, because it may greatly reduce the likelihood of spontaneous delivery. See Chapter 14.

The number of spontaneous deliveries can be increased significantly when there is the will to do so. Motivation to this end depends largely on a clear appreciation of the importance of mothers giving birth to their own children. The solution, as with so much else in labour, is to achieve efficient uterine action. Previous chapters have dealt with how to achieve efficient uterine action during the first stage of labour. Management of the second stage is altered if the urge to push is removed. Improved methods of administration with continuous infusion of low concentration of anaesthetic agent have diminished the importance of this problem. In the absence of an urge to push on diagnosis of full dilatation, one hour is allowed pass before pelvic examination is repeated. If the head has descended to the level of the pelvic floor, pushing is then encouraged. If the head has not descended, oxytocin is infused and pelvic examination is repeated after one hour. Pushing is then commenced for one hour and, if delivery is not imminent, pelvic examination is performed with a view to lift out forceps delivery. The incidence of epidural anaesthesia in primigravidae at this hospital has increased to 15% in 1990, while the incidence of forceps delivery has remained static at 10%.

Case selection

In some centres epidural anaesthesia is *not* given to those who may require it simply because it is not always available, while in other centres epidural anaesthesia **is** given to those who do not require it simply because it is there. Once what has become known as an epidural service has been established and additional personnel employed, there are hidden pressures to increase the head-count merely to justify the existence of the service. Epidural block is available at all times in this hospital, as an integral part of the service, but availability is not a factor which determines its use. A genuine attempt was made to define a role for epidural anaesthesia, and while no claims to scientific accuracy are made because any such study is of necessity based on mainly subjective criteria, the conclusions reached provide a better working guide for mothers and staff than the whims of either party, which so often determine practice elsewhere.

The first conclusion is that epidural anaesthesia has an invaluable contribution to make to the conduct of labour in some primigravidae, but, equally important, that it has little contribution to make to the conduct of labour in multigravidae. The abuse of epidural anaesthesia in multigravidae stems from the mistaken belief that a valid comparison can be drawn between a first and a subsequent labour. A woman who has had an unpleasant first experience of labour, during which she may or may not have had an epidural anaesthetic, frequently seeks a prior commitment on the next occasion because she fears that the experience is likely to be repeated. There are no grounds whatever for such a misapprehension. The obstetrician would serve the interests of the parous woman much better were he to dispel her fears with a simple explanation of the essential difference between a first and a second birth. This course would also save his anaesthetist colleague from the embarrassment of having his efforts to retrieve the prior commitment, entered into by the obstetrician, interrupted by the untimely arrival of the infant, often at dead of night. Moreover, it is in parous women that epidural anaesthesia acts to increase the risk of ruptured uterus, partly because the parous uterus is prone to rupture, and partly because pain has an important protective function in this regard. These are compelling reasons why epidural anaesthesia, in general, should be confined to primigravidae.

The second conclusion is that it is most unwise to enter into a prior commitment, even with a primigravida, because this constitutes a tacit encouragement to a negative, or passive, attitude to childbirth. Prior commitment becomes especially undesirable when it is adopted as a policy to be propagated through antenatal educational channels. There are two sound reasons why an expectant approach to epidural anaesthesia should be practised: first, the reaction of each individual to the actual experience of a first labour can rarely be foretold, perhaps least of all by the woman herself; second, the duration of first labour cannot be predicted. Some 40% of primigravidae deliver themselves within four hours of admission to this hospital, without treatment of any sort, and included in this short timespan is the second stage of labour, when the effects of epidural block are almost wholly adverse. The second stage of labour is tolerated much better than the first, because mothers can exercise an assertive role. Besides, there are not many women who wish to be deprived of the sense of achievement which comes from giving birth to their first child.

Subject to these two strong reservations – that epidural block is confined to primigravidae and that prior commitments are not made – women who derive most benefit from epidural anaesthesia fall into three broad groups, as follows: those who are so disturbed at the very prospect of labour that they are already unduly upset at the point of admission; those who, despite an initial appearance of composure, become unduly upset soon afterwards, and those who are not in sight of delivery six hours later. The number in the first group is related closely to antenatal preparation, the number in the second group to the quality of care after admission, and the number in the third group to the overall duration of labour. Approximately 40% of primigravidae in the National Maternity Hospital qualify for consideration in one or other of these three groups.

With one exception, epidural block is used only for relief of pain. The exception is the occasional woman with an uncontrollable desire to push against a cervix which has not reached full dilatation. Epidural block is not used as a form of therapy in systemic diseases, such as chronic hypertension or pre-eclampsia, or in obstetric abnormalities, such as breech presentation or twins.

Responsibility

The question of ultimate professional responsibility for epidural block deserves more serious consideration than it has yet been given, especially where a prior commitment has been made, or where the person involved is a parous woman. Can it be presumed that the mother, in requesting an epidural anaesthetic, gives blanket acceptance to all the consequences, direct and indirect, without being in a position to fully understand and, therefore, it can reasonably be argued, without fully informed consent? And how far does the obstetrician meet his professional obligation by sanctioning the procedure several months in advance and, therefore, without due regard to the particular circumstances at the time of administration? And what of the anaesthetist summoned to provide an emergency service with little or no knowledge of the background, obstetric or otherwise? Finally, and because timing is so crucial, there is the nurse/midwife whose decision may be of vital importance, particularly in the case of a parous woman. These are issues which do not arise when the decision to use epidural anaesthesia is made on a selective basis during the course of labour.

Summary

Epidural block has a special contribution to make to the management of labour. It should, however, always be treated with due respect. Risks are not confined to the technical procedure itself, but also encompass the patient's ability to respond to shock. The greatly increased need for assisted delivery has a major impact on obstetric practice, although this can be contained by ensuring efficient uterine action. There is the real possibility of rupture of uterus in multigravidae. Epidural block, therefore, should be restricted to primigravidae, given not too early or too late, and never used as a cover for prolonged labour. Prior commitments should not be given. With one exception, epidural block should not be used as a therapeutic agent, but only for relief of pain.

19: Personal Attention

One of the most disturbing prospects of labour is fear of isolation, which the mere mention of a delivery unit seems to engender in many women. This fear of isolation is certainly not a reflection on the standard of medical practice as ordinarily understood; quite the contrary, the problem tends to increase as technical standards rise. The more efficient a unit in strictly medical terms, the more isolated the mothers are likely to feel. The result is that the average citizen seems to have reached the conclusion that medical efficiency and humane considerations are just not compatible. In contemporary obstetrics, to be called efficient has to be regarded as a dubious compliment.

Moral support

Childbirth is a unique event which should provide a sense of profound and lasting satisfaction for mothers, and in which midwives and doctors should count themselves fortunate to share. Yet, as it happens, there are many women who complain bitterly of the apparent indifference of those in whom they placed their trust during the most vulnerable period of their lives. Those closest to the action often do not appear to realise that there are few places on this earth so lonely as a busy delivery unit. As human consciousness is seldom more open to impression than during the momentous hours of labour, a casual approach to just another routine assignment may leave a mother with a burning sense of resentment. Apparently trivial episodes such as a curt tone of voice, a blood-stained glove, a mindless exposure in the indelicate lithotomy position or a failure to convey the result of pelvic examination, though not seemingly of great consequence in themselves, still portray an often deplorable lack of sensitivity in professional staff who should know a great deal better. Because of the heightened sense of awareness at this time, the memory of these affronts to their personal dignity, unintentional though they may be, are nonetheless preserved indefinitely, and in photographic detail, by many women.

The steady emotional decline which is a characteristic feature of labour that is not properly supervised, follows an entirely predictable course. The scenario can be written beforehand. The woman becomes progressively withdrawn from contact with her environment, closes her eyes and buries her face in the pillow, only later to become increasingly restive with contorted features and aimless movements interrupted by frantic outbursts, until eventually a state of panic is reached and self-control is lost completely. Once the morale of a woman in labour has begun to crumble it becomes more and more difficult to restore the balance. Midwives, particularly, must be acutely conscious of the need to keep every woman in labour on a tight emotional rein from the point of her admission until her baby is born, because the further she is allowed to slip down the emotional incline, the more difficult it becomes to recover her composure. Specifically, women in labour must be encouraged to keep their eyes open at all times; closed eyes usually mark the first step along the road to total disintegration. The best protection possible against the gradual erosion of a woman's personal dignity in labour is to hold her attention firmly from the outset.

A sense of panic is a shattering experience from which the individual may never fully recover. This may lead to recurrent nightmares, permanent revulsion to childbirth with consequent marital disharmony, and a sense of antagonism even towards her own child. Not nearly enough attention is paid to this aspect of trauma in childbirth. Panic should rank as one of the most serious complications in obstetrics – more serious than ruptured uterus, in many ways – and it should never be allowed to happen. Much less serious emotional disturbance than this has caused some, albeit misguided, women to advocate a return to home confinement, while freely acknowledging that the purely medical case in favour of hospital confinement remains overwhelming. Consequently, there is a pressing need to recognise that a morbid fear of isolation during labour is widespread, to acknowledge that this fear is only too well founded in practice and to resolve that effective action must be taken to rectify the unfortunate situation.

The nurse/midwife

The only effective antidote to the dread of isolation is a prior guarantee to every expectant mother of continuous personal attention through labour. Personal attention, in this context, means one nurse to one patient, face to face. What personal attention does *not* mean is a group of nurses caring for an equivalent number of patients on a collective basis. Although the total complement of nursing staff deployed in a particular delivery unit may be more than adequate, on paper, still many women continue to complain of being left alone for comparatively long periods. Positive steps are necessary, therefore, to ensure that each woman in labour identifies, by name, with an individual nurse. Although the physical presence of a trained companion is, in itself, a source of considerable comfort to a woman in labour, mere physical presence is not nearly enough. The nurse must appreciate that her primary duty to the mother is to provide the emotional support so desperately needed at this critical time; it is not simply to monitor vital signs in a detached, clinical, manner. The physical condition of the mother must, of course, be supervised, but this is just a matter of recording a few basic items at regular intervals of, say, two hours. These conventional record systems have very little relevance to the great majority of healthy women who are delivered within a few hours of admission. In many centres an altogether disproportionate amount of space on the partograph is allotted to such observations, seemingly to allow for the possibility that every woman might develop fulminating eclampsia or continue in labour for at least 24 hours!

The real value of a personal nurse is best reflected in the facial expression of a woman in labour. Each nurse must purposefully strive to establish a genuine sense of rapport with her charge by seeking to identify everyday topics of common interest. By far the most impressive evidence of the quality of care afforded in a delivery unit is to observe nurse and mother engaged in animated conversation, exchanging smiles in the process. Smiles are more effective than drugs as an antidote to pain. Some are clearly better than others in the field of human relationships, but almost anyone can become proficient when they are trained to be sufficiently aware of the need. A woman's experience of labour depends to a very great extent on the quality of the relationship established with her personal nurse.

The nurse, for her part, derives her greatest satisfaction from the opportunity to contribute so much to one under duress. Those who share moments of great stress tend to forge a lasting bond, and it is truly remarkable how often a woman can recall an individual nurse by name, and her kindness, many years after her first confinement. Naturally communication at this level is much easier to establish in the context of a common culture. Although it is likely to be more difficult when the cultural background of the nurse differs widely from that of her charge, failure to communicate, in any meaningful sense of the word, arises much more often from the nurse not having been taught to appreciate the need. Specifically, every nurse has a responsibility to ensure that the mother genuinely understands the purpose of each medical procedure and the result of each examination, and that she is kept informed of current progress, with a regular review of the time at which her baby is expected to be born.

A prior guarantee is given to every expectant mother who attends this hospital that she will have a personal nurse through the whole of labour, from the point of admission until her baby is born, without regard to the hour of day or night. Many mothers, and observers too, believe this to be the most important development in the conduct of labour in recent years, but they do not always realise that it would not be feasible unless the duration of labour was restricted. The authors rate personal attention as second only in importance to limitation of duration, in management of labour, although the two items are inseparable since one cannot be achieved without the other. With 8,000 deliveries per annum, a personal nurse for every woman in labour is no mean achievement.

The doctor

Doctors must recognise that they too have an indispensable role to play in the provision of personalised care and attention, which is a central issue in good management of labour. The consultant obstetrician, who is ultimately responsible for the welfare of all mothers, must set a clear example because, inevitably, the attitude of the consultant pervades the entire system. Young nurses and doctors follow the example set by their teachers. Unfortunately, on attainment of consultant status, many obstetricians virtually abandon the delivery unit for the antenatal ward or, more likely, the operating theatre, and henceforth, insofar as labour is concerned, their attention is confined to a small cohort of abnormal cases. Even senior registrars are seldom seen in some delivery units until the need for surgical intervention arises. The result is that management of labour in normal women, who represent the overwhelming majority in any given unit, is left to junior residents who have far less experience than senior midwives.

There is absolutely no point in a consultant obstetrician advocating a standard of care and attention to which he is not prepared to make a positive contribution: he must be seen to practise what he preaches. This means that the consultant must be seen in the delivery unit at frequent intervals every day, and he must discuss directly with each expectant mother the questions which he should know to be uppermost in her mind on this momentous occasion. The consultant, in other words, must underwrite the whole ethos of labour management by personal example.

The husband

The extent to which husbands should be influenced to remain with their wives during the entire course of labour and delivery, remains very much an open question. Sometimes it is difficult to avoid the impression that husbands are enlisted to protect their wives against the very fear of isolation which is the subject matter of the present chapter, and sometimes, even, to protect them from unwarranted intervention. Experience in this hospital suggests that women have far more to gain from the presence of a female companion who is not only sympathetic but also well informed and, therefore, in a much better position to provide the type of firm support and guidance which is so sorely needed.

Summary

A personal nurse for every woman in labour has proved a practical proposition in the busiest maternity unit in the British Isles for more than two decades past. Mothers tend to regard this as the most important advance in the conduct of labour in those years. Strict limitation of duration, combined with continuous personal attention, are considered by the authors to be the basic requirements on which a high standard of care in labour ultimately depends. There is close correlation between the two requirements, as neither one is feasible without the other.

20: Role of Doctor

The role of the doctor in the management of labour needs to be considered at four quite different levels of responsibility.

Consultant obstetricians

Consultant obstetricians are in a unique position to influence the standard of care in labour for the better, simply by agreeing a common policy of management within the confines of each institution. The main obstacle to improvement in the quality of care in labour in most institutions is lack of clear direction from the top. Midwives and resident medical officers are frequently placed in the invidious position of having to apply different methods of treatment, in exactly the same clinical circumstances, for no reason other than that the names of the consultants printed on the charts are different. A good illustration of this anomaly is when patients in adjacent beds receive different concentrations of oxytocin or different analgesic drugs, for no more convincing reason than that they happen to have attended the antenatal clinic on different days. The sheer irrationality of this mode of action is a constant affront to the intelligence of professional staff. No one would dare suggest that an intensive care unit in a general hospital could operate efficiently under direction of such a capricious nature. Hence, wherever a genuine wish to improve the quality of care afforded to women in labour exists, the first essential requirement is for the consultant obstetricians to come together and agree to surrender a small portion of their jealously guarded independence for the sake of the common good. This, the authors suggest, is the acid test of goodwill at consultant level. Without this degree of cooperation a delivery unit cannot even begin to achieve its full potential. Naturally, someone must be prepared to take the initial step.

First in order of priority, a chain of command must be sharply defined. There should be one person only in charge of a delivery unit at any given time; a delivery unit cannot operate efficiently under a committee system. For practical purposes the person responsible must be a nurse/midwife. She should be designated as midwife in charge, or Sister, and wear a distinctive uniform which can be recognised instantly by all concerned. Everyone who works in the unit should be subject to her immediate authority. There is no more room for divided responsibility in a delivery unit than there is aboard a ship at sea.

Next, the most sensitive areas of management must be clearly identified and the general outline of procedure standardised. These matters have been addressed in previous chapters under the appropriate headings, as follows: diagnosis, progress, duration, acceleration, etc.

After the critical decision to delegate authority, the most valuable contribution the consultant can make to the conduct of labour is to declare openly full acceptance of responsibility for the outcome. There is no place for equivocation on this issue; delegation of authority on any other terms is meaningless. A bland declaration to the general effect is worthless; subordinate staff need to be convinced that no scapegoat will be sought whenever a mishap occurs – as sooner or later it undoubtedly will as long as humans remain fallible. In practice, unfortunately, this is too often the case. And wherever there is a lack of trust decisions are avoided, treatment is not pursued effectively and caesarean sections are performed, unnecessarily, because surgery provides a soft option for those anxious to avoid being blamed. Contrary to superficial appearances, the decision to commit a woman to caesarean section is taken usually by resident staff before the consultant, who may eventually perform the operation, is even notified.

The consultant obstetrician should be at pains to show equal concern for the composure of all women in labour, and not concentrate his attention on the few who are abnormal. He should be ever conscious of the potential to boost morale by frequent appearances on the 'shop floor'. However, he should not interfere officiously in routine management, but rather encourage the staff to get on with the good work themselves.

Although facilitated greatly by the Mastership system, a high level of cooperation amongst ten consultant obstetricians is a long established feature of this hospital.

Senior registrars

Senior registrars working in this hospital must hold a specialist qualification in obstetrics and gynaecology: they are four in number and there is a strict rule that one must be instantly available, on the premises, at all times. The most important function of the senior registrar is to review the condition of every woman in the delivery unit at regular intervals of four hours approximately, especially late at night. The senior registrar is expected to be on familiar terms with every woman in labour and not, as frequently happens, to remain aloof until summoned to undertake an operative delivery. All but a few obstetric cases are normal at the point of admission, yet many more become abnormal subsequently, simply because they are not supervised properly from the outset. Most complications of labour develop in hospital, and could be readily avoided were proper care and attention to commence at the time of admission. The primary duty of the senior registrar is to ensure that this simple proposition is put into daily practice. A good personal relationship with the midwife in charge is an essential prerequisite to achieve this end.

The senior registrar, in consultation always with the midwife in charge, decides when to terminate labour and also chooses the method of delivery, except in the case of caesarean section which must be referred to the consultant. The need to intervene on the conventional grounds of failure to advance or maternal distress, declines sharply when a policy of active participation is pursued from the outset. The only operative methods of delivery now practised in this hospital are caesarean section and low forceps extraction, with an occasional ventouse; the incidence of these procedures is unusually low by comparison with most other centres. There is no opportunity for trainee specialists to acquire what some might still regard as an essential skill like forceps rotation, because this, like other manoeuvres, is no longer practised. Nowadays, senior registrars are cast firmly in the role of obstetric physicians, rather than surgeons, with most emphasis on the conduct of labour in normal cases.

Residents

Resident medical officers working in this hospital are in the position of training, either as specialists or as family practitioners. None is involved directly in the decision making process. Residents are cast in the role of graduate students whose main purpose is to learn about normal birth; it is assuredly not to teach others how to solve complicated clinical problems of which they themselves have little or no experience. Most young doctors are only too relieved when this situation is frankly acknowledged, because no intelligent young man or woman would wish to be placed in a false position where it is necessary to pretend a level of expertise which he/she, and indeed everyone else, knows he/she does not possess. Those who do not readily accept this position represent a potential hazard to all concerned. Although a resident is on duty in the delivery unit of this hospital at all times – a practical advantage of scale – this is not considered a necessary feature of good practice; indeed, the arrangement could be said to operate more to the personal advantage of the doctor. Residents are always subject to the authority of the midwife in charge and function entirely under her supervision. Practical tasks performed by residents are: artificial rupture of membranes, low forceps extraction and perineal repair. The midwife in charge consults directly with the senior registrar whenever she is in doubt about the management of a particular case. The resident is never in a position to dictate to the midwife nor to overrule her decision in any matter whatsoever.

Medical students

Clinical obstetrics is presented to undergraduates in a manner which is quite different from previous years. Nowadays the aim is purely educational. Undergraduate teaching is based on the assumption that all births take place in hospital, and that comparatively few doctors, therefore, will ever again attend a woman in labour. Nevertheless, it is considered to be one of the fundamental requirements of medical education, in the broadest sense, that every doctor, no matter what discipline he may pursue in later life, should observe at close quarters the nature of childbirth and understand the implications of current management. With this in mind, every student in this medical school must complete eight hours on seven consecutive days in the delivery unit, where he must provide continuous personal care for one mother each day, in a face-to-face relationship. A medical student must function alone, and one student only is permitted in the delivery unit at any given time. Medical students are subject to the same discipline as student midwives. A medical student is not permitted to leave a woman in labour without the express permission of the midwife in charge, and then only when a replacement is immediately available. At the end of seven days the medical student must submit a written report on seven labours conducted under personal supervision, devoting special attention to the emotional impact on the mother, which he has shared.

A medical student may not leave a woman in labour to observe a forceps, twin or breech delivery, even when conducted in an adjoining room. The student is given clearly to understand that the commitment to a woman in labour must be absolute, and that it is the very negation of good obstetric teaching to make use of a woman in labour for one's own advantage, only to abandon her when something more spectacular comes along. This is usually the first, and probably the last, occasion in the whole medical curriculum on which a student comes face to face with a person under severe emotional stress for an extended period of time; it is a salutary experience, one which can be turned to good effect in other branches of medicine. Medical students are immensely gratified to find how much they can contribute by personal commitment in these circumstances. This close encounter with individuals under stress is regarded as the essence of undergraduate teaching on the subject of labour. No longer are medical students exposed to obstetrical curiosities and complicated deliveries· the emphasis is placed on normal birth. It is seen as no function of undergraduate teaching to produce a doctor qualified to commence practice in obstetrics on the day after graduation. A future family practitioner, who may wish to provide antenatal and postnatal care in conjunction with a specialist unit, is required to serve six months as a junior resident in obstetrics after graduation.

Summary

Consultant obstetricians who cannot agree on a common overall policy of management arguably represent the main impediment to improved standards of care in labour. The purpose of this manual is to outline such a policy, and to show how it is put into routine practice in one large teaching centre. To ensure success it is absolutely essential that the role of resident medical officer be redefined as graduate student, and that, as such, he/she be integrated into the obstetric team at the appropriate level. The attention of undergraduates needs to be directed much more to the emotional impact of childbirth and much less to technical procedures which are devoid of educational value.

21: Role of Nurse/Midwife

The role of the nurse/midwife in the management of labour is considered at three levels in this hospital. A Sister, or midwife in charge, and a staff midwife are both state registered general nurses and trained midwives, at different levels of experience. A student midwife is likewise a state registered nurse, having completed three years of vocational training in an accredited general hospital and passed a public examination. Midwifery is a postgraduate subject which requires two additional years of specialist experience and a similar examination. There are 100 student midwives in this hospital at any given time: an intake of 50 per annum. This number constitutes approximately one-half of the entire nursing complement. Wherever the terms nurse and midwife are used in this text they should be regarded as interchangeable, because all are general trained nurses and either trained or trainee midwives.

Sister-in-charge

The Sister, or midwife in charge of the delivery unit, is of paramount importance and it is openly acknowledged that hers is a vital role. In practice she must make all the critical decisions in management which otherwise could go by default: she must confirm or reject the diagnosis of labour in every case admitted; she must measure dilatation of cervix at regular intervals; she must decide when to accelerate progress; and she must carry these decisions into effect – day and night – without reference to medical staff who may be otherwise engaged, if not asleep in bed. Finally, she must decide when the limits of her authority are reached and seek consultation. All this adds up to a formidable responsibility which requires strength of character as well as years of clinical experience.

Whenever the midwife in charge decides that the limits of her authority are reached, the opportunity for consultation with a medical colleague of comparable status is always readily available. It would seem utterly incongruous if a nurse with such wide experience of a highly specialised nature were placed in the position of having to seek the advice of a junior resident with a primary medical qualification. The practical exposure of the average junior resident is restricted to hasty appearances at normal births during a short period of undergraduate residence, possibly instructed by the selfsame nurse.

The midwife in charge of this delivery unit is vested with the authority necessary to perform the duties of her office effectively. Specifically, she does not consult with any doctor below the status of senior registrar. As each midwife in charge is personally responsible for some 1,500 deliveries per annum, she is recognised as an expert in the field, and her advice is keenly sought by members of the medical staff at every level, and on all aspects of labour.

The influence of the midwife in charge is no less important at a humane level. An air of quiet efficiency, which is the hallmark of a good delivery unit, depends on her. This intangible element, which communicates itself so easily to a sensitive observer, is an essential ingredient of the spirit of mutual trust that is such a necessary component of good management. Mothers need to sense that the nurses and doctors to whose care they are committed during these difficult hours behave as members of a team, each with a known part to play. As captain of the team, no one compares with the midwife in charge; so, she surely has the right to expect the unqualified support of colleagues – doctors as well as nurses – in her onerous task. A delivery unit cannot begin to function smoothly without a developed team spirit; everyone suffers when this is lacking.

Five senior midwives with the rank of Sister in charge of delivery unit are employed in this hospital. There is always one on duty, day and night, and only one, to guard against the possible adverse effects of division of responsibility. The result is that each Sister in charge works for an average of one-fifth part of a week: the equivalent of 33 hours and 36 minutes. The actual hours worked are flexible; these are left largely as a matter of mutual agreement. There is no permanent night duty. The Sister in charge of the delivery unit devotes her undivided attention to women in labour. There are no other duties to be performed. She is not responsible for a hospital ward, nor for an operating theatre in the event of caesarean section. She wears a distinctive uniform so that she can instantly be recognised. Without a doubt, her greatest reward is the tremendous sense of job satisfaction which she derives from the ability to make such a worthwhile contribution to the resolution of the perennial problem of stress in labour, on what truly could be described a grand scale. Among the many benefits which have accrued from the practice of active management of labour, none is more gratifying to observe than the boost given to the professional status of midwives in this hospital.

Staff midwife

A staff midwife acts as personal assistant to the Sister in charge of the delivery unit and is responsible directly to her. Two staff midwives are present at all times and their hours of duty correspond with those of the Sister in charge. A staff midwife, like a Sister in charge, acts mainly in a supervisory capacity and in normal circumstances is not identified with an individual mother. At least one trained midwife is present at every delivery, and most deliveries are conducted without any reference to medical staff.

Student midwife

Four student midwives complete a team. A student midwife plays a different role. She provides continuous support for one woman through labour. The role ensures that she soon comes to appreciate that a nurse's unique contribution to the conduct of labour is made at personal level. This requires that far more attention be paid to a woman's face than to her abdomen, or to her vital signs. As this is a midwifery training school, students perform these duties under constant supervision; they would be suitable for trained personnel otherwise.

The procedure is as follows: the mother is admitted to the delivery unit by a student midwife who remains with her during labour, conducts her delivery, presents her newborn infant and, eventually, accompanies her to the postnatal ward. This ideal is not always realised fully because it is affected by hours of duty, but as labour rarely lasts longer than eight hours it applies in most cases. It is very seldom that more than two nurses are involved, consecutively, with the same woman. Each nurse keenly appreciates that her primary duty is to sustain her charge's flagging spirits during the tedious hours of the first stage, and then to encourage her to achieve spontaneous delivery through her own efforts, in the second stage. Student midwives spend six months, out of the total period of two years required for midwifery training, in the delivery unit.

General principles

The personal nurse is instructed to sit always in front of, and in direct eye contact with, a recumbent mother. She must not stand over her, in a dominant position, and never behind, out of her line of vision. A comfortable seat is provided for this purpose. Should a woman prefer to walk, her nurse accompanies her.

Nurses are encouraged to develop close personal relationships with mothers, and to converse with them freely on any subject which holds their interest, thus distracting attention from the labour predicament. In our experience, young, properly motivated girls perform this task with remarkable success when they are made sufficiently conscious of the need, and given the right example by their superiors. Nurses are taught that women in labour have a natural tendency to withdraw from contact with their surroundings and turn inwards on themselves, and that this inclination to introspection is exaggerated greatly by analgesic drugs. They are forewarned about the woman who closes her eyes, buries her face in the pillow and continues to complain even between contractions. They know that these are signs which indicate that the thread of personal contact is being eroded and that, once broken, it will be very difficult to mend. They are acutely sensitive to the fact that a woman who turns her back, is passing a devastating judgment on the quality of the nursing care.

The two subjects of conversation which are of abiding interest to a woman in labour are the expected time of delivery and the welfare of her unborn child. A good nurse appreciates the need for constant reassurance that steady progress is being made and that the baby is likely to be born soon. This information should be instantly demonstrable on any worthwhile partograph. Hopefully, the partograph will have been thoroughly explained beforehand, at antenatal classes, with this important sequel in mind. In that case, mothers can be expected to take a keen interest in the medical proceedings. A partograph which does not fulfil this simple predictive function has forfeited much of its value.

Specific duties

The personal nurse has specific clinical duties to perform at regular intervals during labour. She must record the mother's pulse, temperature, respirations, blood pressure and urine, as well as the fetal heart and liquor. In the event of oxytocin being used, she must regulate the rate of infusion and enter each contraction as it occurs. As a student, she works under close supervision and must report any untoward event to her immediate superior.

Summary

No form of management of labour can be really effective unless it can be practised by nurses independently, almost, of doctors. This requires a level of mutual confidence between nurses and doctors which is not too often found. A clear chain of command, which can be seen to function with military efficiency but with a human face, is an essential requirement. Nurses and doctors must come to appreciate that much more can be contributed to emotional equilibrium than to physical survival in circumstances where 95% of maternity cases are normal at the point of admission. One of the most impressive features of active management of labour is the sense of purpose which it gives to all levels of the midwifery profession in a busy delivery unit.

22: Role of Mother

It could be too easily overlooked that mothers themselves have the most important contribution of all to make to the birth process. No matter how high the quality of care on offer from nurses and doctors, the entire experience may well prove disastrous when the mother is not properly prepared. Therefore, a serious obligation rests on expectant mothers to take full advantage of the educational facilities available, so as to learn the nature of their role and how best this can be fulfilled. Mothers should not be allowed – any more than nurses or doctors are allowed – to evade their responsibilities in this matter. They should be disabused of the notion that nurses and doctors can be expected to cope with the inevitable turmoil, as part of their normal duties. Paternalism is not to be considered a virtue here; an expectant mother should be made face the fact that the birth of her child is primarily her responsibility.

All this is to presume that adequate educational facilities are both readily available and relevant in content. First and foremost, what is taught must be seen to correspond with everyday practice in the institution. It is not just teachers who must be credible; nurses and doctors also must know exactly what women have been taught to expect, prior to admission. If more than lip service is to be paid to the proposition that education is a necessary component of an obstetric service with pretensions to optimal standards of care in labour, then classes must cease to be regarded as optional extras, conducted by teachers who are far removed from clinical practice and virtually ignored by those in positions of greatest influence. The most important element in the entire educational process is, of course, education to the need for education: only clinicians are in a position to impress this on their charges. It is much too late to begin education in a labour ward.

Every adult woman must, in the final analysis, be made to feel the proper custodian of her personal well-being, not to mention that of her child. Labour is no exception to this general rule. An expectant mother owes it to herself, her husband and her child, and every other woman sharing the facilities of the same delivery unit, to be well briefed on the subject of a mother's contribution to labour. The disruptive effect of one disorganised and frightened woman in a delivery unit extends far beyond her individual comfort and safety, and there should be no hesitation in telling her so.

Mothers also have a duty to those who care for them during labour. The reciprocal nature of this compact deserves much more emphasis than it is given. Where necessary, it should be bluntly stated that nurses are not expected to submit themselves to the sometimes outrageous conduct of perfectly healthy women who cannot be persuaded to cross a narrow corridor from an antenatal clinic. Such women must learn how to behave with dignity and purpose during the most important event of their lives. Nor should nurses be held responsible for the degrading scenes which occasionally result from failure of a woman to fulfil her part of the compact.

Women who have participated in the educational programme of this hospital generally portray a high level of insight into the essential features of the birth process. They understand the need for professional confirmation of their provisional diagnosis of labour, they know that subsequent progress is measured in terms of opening of the neck of the womb and, when progress is slow, they appreciate that it makes good sense to take corrective action at the proper time. All this is evident from the partograph with which they are already quite familiar. It is hardly surprising, therefore, that women in labour often request acceleration with oxytocin when it becomes clear that satisfactory progress is not being made. By way of contrast, they need to be convinced whenever the question of induction is mooted.

Suggestions that women in some other centres regard oxytocin with suspicion and, in the event of slow progress, frequently decline acceleration, could only be the result of misunderstandings which, in turn, reflect poorly on the quality of the educational service. Paradoxically, induction rates, which involve identical procedures, may be close to 50% in these same centres. The authors never cease to be impressed by the ability of the average woman to assimilate the essential facts about labour when these are properly presented.

Summary

Expectant mothers deserve to be treated as adults and made fully aware that childbirth is primarily their responsibility. However, they must be provided with adequate educational services so that they can learn how to achieve their goal. Obstetricians must realise that few mature women really want to be treated like irresponsible children on this momentous occasion.

23: Care of Fetus

Overall care of the fetus during labour is based on the simple premise that the fetus who presents as a case of hypoxia during the course of normal labour is almost sure to have been embarrassed before labour began. The occasional exception is likely to be the result of an accident of labour, which causes acute hypoxia in a hitherto normal fetus: prolapse of cord is the classical example. The aims, therefore, are two-fold: first, to identify the fetus who is already embarrassed and, second, to ensure that the labour itself remains normal.[12]

Artificial rupture of membranes

To identify the fetus who is already embarrassed, artificial rupture of membranes is performed as soon as a formal diagnosis of labour is made and the woman is, therefore, committed to delivery. A free flow of clear liquor is regarded as a virtual guarantee that the function of the placenta is sufficient to withstand the pressures of normal labour. The opportunity is taken to exclude prolapse of cord. A sample of liquor is retained in a test tube for further inspection in every case.

This procedure is intended to identify cases which have escaped detection in late pregnancy, before the additional stress of labour can cause an already precarious balance to deteriorate abruptly.

Meconium

Meconium is regarded as a clinical sign of great potential significance. At the outset, women in labour are divided into two groups: 90% with clear liquor and 10% with meconium. The division into low risk and high risk cases is made on this simple evidence which is of fetal origin, and not on whether the mother suffers from pre-eclampsia, for example, or had her last menstruation 42 weeks previously.

Not all meconium, however, is accorded the same significance. There is a world of difference between light meconium staining of a large volume of liquor, and meconium that is virtually undiluted, with umbilical cord, membranes and even endometrium coloured green through its entire depth when exposed subsequently at caesarean section.

Meconium is interpreted as evidence of placental insufficiency of some duration, not as evidence of short term fetal distress. Moreover, meconium seldom appears for the first time during the course of normal labour.

Three grades of meconium are recognised, as follows:

Grade I   A good volume of liquor stained lightly with meconium.
Grade II   A reasonable volume of liquor with a heavy suspension of meconium.

Grade III Thick meconium which is undiluted and resembles sieved spinach.

All grades of meconium must be reported to the senior registrar. A wide margin of discretion is permitted in Grade I; after careful review of all the clinical circumstances no further action is taken in most cases. A fetal blood sample is mandatory in Grade II; treatment is determined largely by the result. Caesarean section is performed in Grade III unless an easy vaginal delivery is imminent; not only hypoxia but also meconium inhalation is a real possibility here.

No liquor

Failure to recover any liquor whatsoever, at artificial rupture of membranes is, for reasons of safety, treated as meconium Grade II, although clear liquor frequently appears at a later stage.

Fetal heart

Direct auscultation of the fetal heart is a duty performed by the personal nurse who supervises each labour. This is for one full minute, at intervals of 15 minutes during the first stage, and after each contraction during the second stage.

Blood sample

Fetal acidosis is accepted as the definitive test for hypoxia. Only in exceptional circumstances is a woman subjected to caesarean section for the indication fetal distress without this confirmation. In practice, this situation is likely to arise most frequently in the presence of Grade II meconium, where caesarean section would have to be performed – sometimes unnecessarily – were the definitive test not available.

Electronic monitors

Electronic monitors play no part in routine care in this hospital, but, in the event of a blood sample being taken because of clinical evidence of distress – most likely in the form of meconium at rupture of membranes – a scalp electrode is applied before the result is available. This provides a continuous record between definitive blood tests in suspect cases, but it would be highly improbable that the tracing alone would determine treatment.

Because of the long running controversy concerning the respective values of continuous electronic monitoring and intermittent auscultation, a decision was made to compare the two methods in the context of the practice of this hospital. Arising from this, a prospective randomised trial of unprecedented scope was undertaken by our colleague Dr MacDonald in conjunction with the National Perinatal Epidemiology Unit in the

United Kingdom, between March 1981 and April 1983. Certain cases were specifically excluded from the trial beforehand: those with meconium or no liquor at rupture of membranes; these represented 6% of the total. All other cases were included, without regard to risk status by conventional standards such as pre-eclampsia, antepartum haemorrhage, diabetes, etc. The number of eligible cases was 12,964 of which 6,474 were allocated, on a random basis, to the electronically monitored group and 6,490 to the intermittently auscultated group. Both methods were supported by fetal blood samples as the need arose.

The results showed no difference in perinatal mortality rate: there were 14 deaths in each group. Neither was there a significant difference in Apgar scores, need for intubation, or admission to the Special Care Baby Unit. There was one significant difference: the incidence of neonatal convulsions in those who survived. There were nine cases of neonatal convulsions in the electronically monitored group, compared with 21 in the intermittently auscultated group. When these 30 infants were examined after 12 months, six showed evidence of permanent damage, all of the cerebral palsy type: three were from the electronically monitored group and three were from the intermittently auscultated group. The balance, in other words, had been restored.[13,14] See also Chapter 28.

Significantly, the perinatal mortality rate in cases excluded from the trial on the basis of meconium or no liquor, was five times greater than the overall figure for cases included. The caesarean section rate was low and not significantly different in either group: 2.4 and 2.2%, respectively. Elective caesarean sections are, of course, not represented here. The close similarity between the two groups is almost certainly the result of retaining the blood sample as the final arbiter of distress in both instances. There can be little doubt that electronic monitors, without the benefit of blood tests as control, lead to a sharp increase in the caesarean section rate for the indication fetal distress.

Normal labour

Since the contention is that normal placental function is sufficient to sustain the fetus through the exigencies of normal labour, it is necessary to have a clear understanding of what is meant by this term. Labour is defined as normal when delivery is effected within 12 hours through the efforts of the mother, although this need not preclude use of low forceps. Steps taken to ensure that labour conforms to this definition of normality would appear to be a valuable contribution to the welfare of the fetus also. Trauma is to be avoided at all costs, and trauma is much less likely to occur when mothers deliver themselves.

Summary

A fetus who enters labour in good condition is well-equipped by nature to withstand the challenge of normal birth. Routine supervision in this hospital is based on simple clinical evidence meticulously observed. Particular attention is paid to meconium present at the outset. This test is universally available and needs no specialised equipment or techniques. Electronic monitors represent an alternative method of routine supervision of the fetal heart, but they do not improve results. In either event, a fetal blood sample can serve to reduce the caesarean section rate for the indication fetal distress.

24: Induction

This manual is not concerned with induction as a separate entity but only indirectly, in so far as it may impinge on management of labour. The relationship was discussed briefly in Chapter 2, in which two points were made with special emphasis: first, that there should be no confusion between induction and acceleration of labour and, second, that induction has a profoundly adverse effect on management of labour as a whole. Furthermore, the adverse effects of induction are by no means confined to the individuals directly involved: they extend to affect everyone delivered in a hospital in which induction is freely practised. Against this background, there are three different aspects of the subject which merit close attention: indications for induction, suitability for induction, and methods of induction.[15]

Indications

The laxity, or otherwise, of the indications for induction, determines the magnitude of the iatrogenic problem created by this form of medical intervention, in each institution. One of many unfortunate consequences of an uncritical application of statistics to obstetric practice in recent years has been to expand the indications for induction to encompass almost all births. Pre-eclampsia and prolonged pregnancy are the two outstanding examples; these are the indications for induction recorded in a large majority of cases, whether the incidence be high or low. While it is true that both pre-eclampsia and prolonged pregnancy are associated with a significant increase in perinatal mortality, this applies only when diastolic pressure exceeds 100 mmHg or duration of pregnancy exceeds 42 weeks. The relevant statistics have been widely misinterpreted with the result that a high proportion of all cases on whom induction is performed for pre-eclampsia or prolonged pregnancy – or other equally vague category – do not conform to any critical standards. Furthermore, even in the minority of cases who do conform to critical standards, the likelihood of an unfavourable outcome is so small that it does not justify a routine approach, where many are subjected to a potentially hazardous form of treatment in the hope that a few might benefit. Induction of labour, so called, is undertaken far too often on a rule of thumb basis with little attempt to select the individuals who are genuinely in need of deliverance.

In this hospital, indications for induction have become increasingly selective, particularly in pre-eclampsia and postmaturity, which together account for the bulk of reported cases almost everywhere. Induction is now seldom performed for pre-eclampsia, unless in addition to hypertension there is also proteinuria, or for postmaturity, unless there is objective evidence of impaired placental function as shown by reduced liquor volume at 42 weeks. The conclusion is that the rate of induction overall should not exceed 10%; this represents a total of about 700 cases annually.

Suitability

The standard of suitability adopted largely determines the number of failures. As the indication for delivery is seldom absolute, the decision to proceed with induction should be subject to the likelihood of success in each instance. Induction is not attempted in this hospital unless the head is engaged and the cervix is, at the very least, reasonably favourable. Whenever the need to terminate pregnancy arises before these basic conditions are fulfilled, caesarean section is performed on the grounds that induction is not the correct method of treatment in these circumstances. Prostaglandin, to ripen the cervix, is rarely used. Attention is drawn to the low caesarean section rate in spite of this seemingly radical approach.

An implication that the end justifies the means in this context, and that whatever transpires subsequently can be blamed on the condition for which the induction was nominally performed, is not tenable. In all walks of life prudence requires that no action be taken without due consideration of possible consequences; this is certainly true of obstetrics. The decision to interrupt the course of pregnancy is a clear example of a balance of risks. The choice of induction as the method of achieving this end may be quite correct in one instance, where conditions are favourable, but wholly incorrect in another, where conditions are unfavourable. Far too many inductions are undertaken for dubious reasons in unfavourable circumstances, with the result that the treatment is more dangerous than the, often nebulous, disease. An uncritical approach to this potentially serious issue is the cause of considerable disquiet, which is not confined to obstetricians.

Method

The method of induction determines the length of time spent in a delivery unit by women who are not yet in labour. This consideration has some important consequences, both for those individuals directly involved and for all the other women who must share the facilities of a delivery unit where there is a large number of inductions. To reduce time spent in the delivery unit by women not yet in labour – primarily in their own interest, but also in the general interest – the method of induction used in this hospital consists of simple amniotomy. The final decision to proceed with amniotomy is taken at pelvic examination by a doctor with the status of senior registrar. The forewaters are ruptured in a special location and at a fixed time of day, and the woman returns to the antenatal ward to await the onset of labour. Meanwhile, no restrictions are placed on her movements. The result is that 90% of women subjected to amniotomy for the purpose of induction are already in labour when they first enter the delivery unit. Subsequent progress is similar in all respects to that of women admitted from their homes, whether this is expressed in terms of hours spent in the delivery unit, drugs administered for relief of pain or operative procedures undertaken.

Labour does not begin within 24 hours of amniotomy in 10% of cases; these are recorded as failed inductions. Next morning, they are transferred to the delivery unit where oxytocin is given as a back-up procedure. The same solution as for acceleration of labour is used: 10 units in 1 litre of 5% dextrose. The maximum rate of infusion is 60 drops per minute and 1 litre only is allowed. The result is that 90% of these exceptional cases, already classified as failed inductions because they did not respond to simple amniotomy, deliver vaginally within 12 hours. Caesarean section is performed when labour is not well advanced after 1 litre – which requires six hours – or, in any event, after a woman has been 12 hours in the delivery unit.

This method of procedure ensures that only one in every 100 admissions to the delivery unit of this hospital receives oxytocin for the purpose of induction. In numerical terms this means, say, 70 women out of a total of 7,000 on an annual basis. The contribution made by this simple arrangement to the overall quality of care afforded to the totality of women in labour is enormous. Facilities, especially in terms of human resources, are not dissipated in the care of women who are not in labour and who, therefore, should not be in a delivery unit. There are many delivery units in which at any given time, one in every two women is not in labour. Nonetheless, these are the very women who attract most attention, and for a much longer time. This attention can only be made available at the expense of the women who are in labour.

The main argument advanced in support of the immediate use of oxytocin, after amniotomy, to induce labour, is based on the fact that the likelihood of infection increases with the passage of time, between amniotomy and delivery: the induction–delivery interval. In practice, however, the risk is small when cases are carefully selected and delivery is almost sure to take place within 24 hours. Under these circumstances, the risk of infection is certainly not sufficient to justify serious disruption of an entire delivery service by the admission of a large number of women who are not in labour. This is a good example of the balance of risks applied to a much wider issue.

Summary

The impact of an institutional policy which invokes a high rate of induction cannot be evaluated in isolation. It is not sufficient to examine the immediate results of the procedure itself; the indirect effects on other aspects of hospital practice must also be taken into account. The adverse effects of a high rate of induction on the overall management of labour are so great that it might reasonably be argued that the most effective single contribution to improved standards of care in such an institution, would be a virtual embargo on this procedure. As a complete embargo is hardly a practical proposition, induction should be regarded as a necessary evil, to be restricted to a small number of individuals in which the indication is genuine and the conditions are favourable. The method should be chosen to cause least disturbance to the individual and least disruption to the entire delivery service. Unquestionably, simple amniotomy is that method: one woman in 100 receives oxytocin to induce labour in this hospital.

25: Organisation

Although there may be other fields of medical practice of which it could be said with equal truth that more is to be gained from sound organisational methods than from sophisticated techniques, there can be few more obvious examples than a modern delivery unit. No matter how sophisticated the equipment may become, a delivery unit cannot begin to function properly unless the basic organisation is sound.[16]

Delivery units, in general, suffer from poor organisational standards mainly because they lack central direction; in terms of management they often border on the chaotic:—unable to cope with occasional additional pressures even though they are overstaffed for most of the time. Corporate spirit tends to be poorly developed, with nurses, doctors and even administrators failing to cooperate closely with each other, sometimes within the same group. Sometimes they are actually in open conflict. Inevitably, this situation operates to the detriment of the consumers.

Better organisation can, quite literally, transform the quality of care afforded to all women in labour; in addition, it can greatly enhance the level of job satisfaction of nurses, and provide an objective basis for costs incurred in a very expensive service. As is so often the case, good practice corresponds with good economics in this instance. Both make good sense.

Nursing services

In terms of organisation, the key to the solution of the problems of a modern delivery unit lies in the nursing service. Nursing staff must be deployed for the declared purpose of providing professional attention at personal level for every woman in labour. The same number of nurses, of equal status, must operate day and night, as concrete evidence of the fact that the welfare of mothers and infants is not to be influenced by the time at which a birth happens to occur. This cannot be achieved through a haphazard approach: careful planning is needed.

Scale

A large scale operation confers an obvious advantage in this respect because it helps to eliminate peaks and valleys in terms of numbers of babies born at different hours of day, days of week, or seasons of year. In this hospital, presently with some 7,000 deliveries per annum, the percentage of total births which occur in each of the 8-hour periods corresponding with official working shifts, falls between 30 and 35, and in each month, between 7.5 and 9.5. This provides a reasonably even distribution at all times. Furthermore, large scale permits a nucleus of highly skilled midwives to be employed on a wholetime commitment to the delivery unit, so that they are neither required to divide their attention with antenatal or postnatal wards, nor to leave women in labour to assist at caesarean sections.

Intensive care

Nowadays, delivery units are frequently spoken of in the context of intensive care, although services, especially nursing services, continue to function in a largely fragmentary manner, devoid of any rational explanation and heavily concentrated in daylight hours. This, it would appear, is to suit staff rather than 'patients'. There is a wide credibility gap here that needs to be closed.

Bottleneck

In every maternity hospital the delivery unit represents a bottleneck through which all mothers must pass. Hence, it is here that the number of confinements for which it is possible to cater in the entire system is determined. Accommodation elsewhere, especially in postnatal wards which comprise the bulk of obstetrical beds, is extremely flexible. The immediate effect of a general reduction of stay in a postnatal ward by one day, would be to increase the functional capacity of a maternity hospital by at least 20%. These are considerations of great practical importance in terms of public expenditure at current levels. In a maternity service, only a special care baby unit can compare with a delivery unit in terms of concentration of skill, with corresponding costs. Both should be efficiently used. Antenatal and postnatal wards are areas of comparatively low level care where most mothers can, and indeed should, fend largely for themselves.

Duration of stay

The newfound ability to limit the duration of stay and, therefore, quantify the total number of consumer hours to be serviced, has transformed the previously haphazard approach to planning in this area. To take a simple example: one nurse in the course of her working day can supervise one woman during a labour which lasts 8 hours, whereas three nurses are required to supervise the same woman during a labour which lasts 24 hours. The problem is further compounded by extensive use of induction, where nurses are engaged in looking after women who, for much of the time at least, are not in labour. A liberal attitude towards induction constitutes an almost insurmountable barrier to the application of sound organisational methods in a delivery unit, especially where the central issue of nursing services is concerned.

The practice

There were 6,328 babies born in the National Maternity Hospital during 1991. The total nursing complement employed whole-time in the delivery unit was 38, of which number 18 were graduate and 20 were student midwives. This complement includes provision for holiday relief and other off-duty situations such as study leave and occasional illness.

There was no other category of nursing attendant involved. Hence, the average number of babies born for each nurse employed was 167. This compares with 207 in 1970, when 6,225 babies were born. The latter figure was the subject of a report in Proceedings of the Royal Society of Medicine, where comparison was made with an average figure of 84 births for each nurse employed in the delivery unit, in a sample of five similar institutions around the British Isles. The unit cost of production, relating salaries paid to nurses to number of babies born, was three times higher in the other centres, although the level of remuneration was comparable. Paradoxically, this was the only one of the six units surveyed where a personal nurse was provided for every woman in labour

Nurses work 8-hour shifts. The number of nurses on duty in the delivery unit at all times is seven: one Sister, two staff midwives and four student midwives. There are five delivery rooms. To ensure that everyone in labour has continuous personal attention one student is allotted to each room. Staff midwives act mainly in a supervisory capacity, with the Sister in complete overall charge. A Sister or staff midwife employed in the delivery unit works for 33 hours 36 minutes and a student for 40 hours each week. Hence the unit cost of production, in which nurses' salaries are by far the largest item, can be readily estimated. This provides a basis of comparison from year to year and between one institution and another. Due to a steady decline in total births from a peak of 8,964 in 1981, the number of deliveries per nurse employed has now fallen well below the critical figure of 200.

Although none is nearly as important as the nursing element, there are other aspects of the comprehensive organisational requirement of an efficient delivery service which, hopefully, may have been discerned as a continuous thread running through the pages of this text. Most important is the need for central direction to draw the diverse elements together, thus welding a team out of a collection of individuals of various disciplines and different levels of seniority. The result should be an efficient, happy and economical unit which is seen to make sense to all who work there.

Summary

The ideal combination of a nucleus of highly skilled midwives with continuous personal attention for every woman in labour, is feasible only in a busy unit where a limit is set to duration and everyone receives individual attention simply because it is needed for a shorter length of time. However, it would be naive to assume that this situation could be achieved overnight, or that it is simply a matter of opting for the appropriate technical procedures. In the final analysis, good organisation is more advantageous to labour management than any number of sophisticated techniques.

26: Cervix in Labour

Obstetrics suffers grievously from lack of accurate definition, not only of common clinical conditions, of which labour itself is a prime example, but even of terms commonly used to describe essential features of these conditions. One suspects that if several individuals who worked in the same delivery unit, and who had long grown accustomed to exchange these mundane terms on a daily basis, were asked what precisely they understood the words 'effacement' and 'dilatation' to mean or, better still, were presented with pencil and paper and asked to reproduce them as simple line drawings, the results would be very different. Yet few would dispute that it is a matter of considerable practical consequence that there should be, at the very least, a common language amongst workers in the same field.

Parity factor

Time and again, in preceding chapters, attention has been drawn to the need to consider primigravidae and multigravidae as if they belonged to different biological species in all matters relating to labour. The cervix is one more example. To the examining finger, the primigravid cervix and the multigravid cervix are so widely dissimilar that they could well be different organs. The greatest divergence concerns the external os which remains permanently ajar after the birth of a first child. Herein lies a source of endless confusion. Hence, the parity factor must be taken into account whenever the terms effacement and dilatation are under consideration. The best way to illustrate this statement is by diagrammatic representation:

The nulliparous cervix is tubular in shape; although constricted somewhat at either end, both internal os and external os usually allow a finger-tip to pass.

The parous cervix is tent-like in shape; the internal os is of comparable size but the external os hangs loose to the extent that it may allow two fingers, or possibly more, to pass.

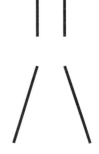

Effacement

Effacement refers to the process of inclusion of the entire length of cervical canal into the lower segment, or body, of uterus. This begins at the internal os and proceeds downwards to the external os, at which level effacement is complete. The process of effacement is not tied to a particular time schedule: it may occur late in pregnancy or be delayed in its entirety until labour begins. An important corollary is that effacement of cervix is not an essential requirement for a diagnosis of labour: a woman may be in labour without her cervix being effaced, much less dilated. Hence, the practical importance of a 'show' or spontaneous rupture of membranes, as discussed in Chapter 5. However, in the event of effacement not having taken place at least to some extent beforehand, duration of labour is likely to be prolonged. These are usually the troublesome cases.

Dilatation

Dilatation refers to the external os only. The external os cannot begin to open until the process of effacement is complete. Effacement and dilatation are consecutive, not simultaneous events. This sequential relationship is of paramount importance: a cervix which is not effaced cannot possibly be dilated, even though, as is often the case in a parous woman, the external os may freely admit two fingers at pelvic examination. The patulous state of the external os in a parous woman is a relict of a previous birth; it is passive in nature and must not be confused with the active process of dilatation which denotes labour here and now. Naturally, therefore, by the time a parous cervix achieves full effacement it is already the equivalent of 2 cm open on the dilatation scale.

Transition

The point of transition, where effacement ends and dilatation begins, requires special attention. At this point the presence or absence of painful uterine contractions is decisive. Since without painful uterine contractions there is no question of a woman being in labour, a fully effaced cervix in these circumstances should be said to admit one or more fingers, as the case may be, whereas with painful uterine contractions the same cervix should be said to be dilated to the extent of 1 cm or more. The former expression is intended to convey an inert or static situation; the latter is intended to convey an evolving or dynamic situation. At a practical level, the issue is straightforward: should an individual who believes herself to be in labour be retained in the delivery unit, with the almost inevitable consequence that she is committed to delivery, perhaps ultimately by caesarean section? Since one caesarean section may well lead to another, a woman's subsequent lifestyle may be significantly altered as a result of this decision, hence the need for close attention to detail in this pivotal area.

(1)   (2)

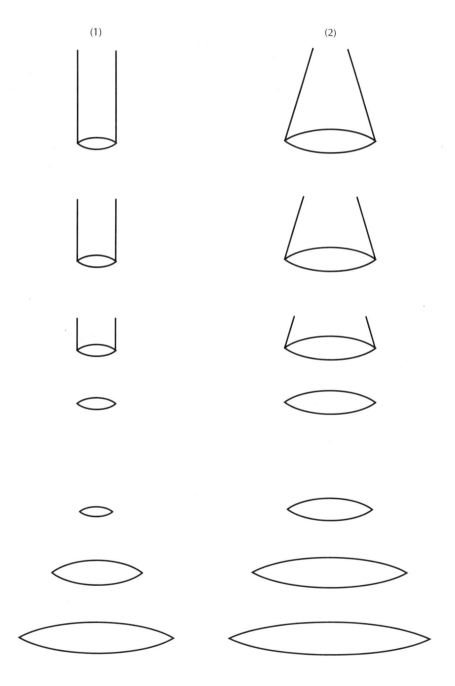

Figure 2 Diagrammatic representation of process of effacement followed by dilatation of primigravid (1) and multigravid (2) cervix.

Summary

There is not nearly sufficient appreciation of the fact that very many of the problems encountered in a delivery unit have their origin in wrong diagnosis. Unwittingly, these are classified as dystocia, or one of its three components: inefficient uterine action, posterior position or cephalopelvic disproportion. Given the fundamental importance of diagnosis, therefore, and of the central role of the cervix in the decision making process, surprisingly little attention is directed to the perceived meaning of the terms used to describe the sequence of events at this critical juncture. Instead, the terms effacement and dilatation tend to be taken for granted and quickly glossed over, as if everybody understood precisely what is meant. As always, the need for verbal precision is greatest in doubtful cases where diagnosis presents a genuine problem; no problem exists when the cervix is well dilated and these cases give rise to few difficulties during the subsequent course of labour, in any event.

27: Caesarean Section Rates

From the maternal aspect of childbirth, surely the most striking change in the practice of obstetrics over the past 25 years is the explosive growth of caesarean section, almost worldwide. Thus, the caesarean birth rate across the USA has increased almost sixfold – from 5% to 30% – between 1965 and 1990, representing a numerical increase from 150,000 to 1,000,000 annually. In the process, caesarean section has achieved the dubious distinction of becoming the most frequently performed hospital operation of any category in North America, relegating hysterectomy, perhaps not without a tinge of irony, into second place in the national surgical league table.

Similar trends have been reported from Canada, Latin America, Australia, most of Europe and Scandinavia and increasingly, from less developed countries which are open to Western influence. Whether calculated in terms of human anxiety and discomfort, or in terms of surgical and anaesthetic complications – which although usually minor, are sometimes major and occasionally fatal – or in purely monetary terms, the cost is truly enormous.[17]

Sense of proportion

In the light of this extraordinary increase in the number of women who are subjected to major abdominal operations which are of no direct benefit to themselves, the detached observer might reasonably assume that the benefits conferred on their offspring could be shown to be overwhelming. Alas, this is far from being the case. Indeed Pearson, writing in the American Journal of Obstetrics and Gynecology in January 1984, described the phenomenon as the greatest uncontrolled medical experiment of our time. As justification for the increase in caesarean section rates must be sought in improved perinatal results, the Tables presented in Section III of this manual are of particular interest; similar information is not always readily available from other sources. Briefly, the Tables show that although the caesarean section rate has not changed substantially over 25 years in this hospital, the perinatal mortality rate has continued to decline steadily over the same period. These figures provide a basis for comparison with other centres.

An increase of just 1% in the caesarean section rate at this hospital would entail about 70 additional operations; 5%, 350 additional operations; and 10%, 700 additional operations, on an annual basis. At a practical level this latter figure means that more than two additional caesarean sections would be performed on each day of the year. As many would be at irregular hours, this would create a logistical problem of major proportions which could be resolved only to the detriment of other features of the service. And still the caesarean section rate would hardly exceed 15%, a figure which seems perfectly acceptable in many comparable establishments. So much for the mother: what of the child?

In 1990 there were 81 perinatal deaths, over 500 g, in this hospital (12.8/1000) of which 23 were attributed to lethal congenital malformations.

Amongst 58 normal infants (9.1/1000), eight died during labour (1.2/1000) and 19 within 28 days after birth (3/1000). Eleven of these neonatal deaths occurred in infants born before 28 weeks gestation, while six of the remaining eight infants weighed less than 2,500 g. Neonatal convulsions occurred in 10 infants (1.6/1000); subsequent examinations suggest that five are normal, four are abnormal, and one was lost to follow up. Chapter 28 deals with the critically important subject of cerebral palsy in this hospital.

Impact of neonatology

The overall reduction in perinatal mortality in recent years coincided with the emergence of neonatology as a major speciality, thus leading to the present position where given a normal infant, born alive without hypoxia or trauma after 28 weeks in a tertiary care centre, is almost sure to survive and develop satisfactorily. The very success of neonatologists has resulted in subtle pressure being brought to bear on obstetricians to dispense with the whole troublesome process of labour altogether. This would seem a perfectly reasonable proposition were there only one patient to be considered. But, unfortunately, in obstetrics there are two, and while no one would dispute the contention that babies have a right to be well born, experience compiled in this hospital over an extended period shows that comparable results can be achieved by far less intrusive means. Whenever the occasion arises, therefore, it is a matter of utmost importance that facile conclusions in respect of cause and effect relationships between caesarean section rates and perinatal mortality rates, much less morbidity rates, should be vehemently challenged; otherwise, it is not inconceivable that, eventually, nearly all babies will be born by caesarean section, if only because obstetricians are forced into a position of having to protect themselves from charges of malpractice. Mothers will be the losers if obstetricians renege on the dual responsibility which is the distinctive feature of their speciality (Figure 3).

Indications

The National Institutes of Health Consensus Development Report on Cesarean Childbirth[18] clearly identified dystocia, or abnormal labour, as the main reason for the rapid expansion of caesarean section in the USA. Dystocia accounted for one-half of all primary operations and, by inference therefore, for approximately the same proportion of repeat procedures. The consistently low caesarean rate in this hospital can be explained almost entirely by the corresponding figure for dystocia. The caesarean rate for dystocia alone in the USA exceeds the caesarean rate for all indications in Dublin. There are some differences under other headings, such as fetal distress and breech presentation, but these are small by comparison. Ultimately, the caesarean rate in a given population is determined by the management of labour in first time mothers with vertex presentation and single fetus; that is what this book is about. Parous women do not suffer from dystocia to any significant extent.

121

Table 27.1. Indications for caesarean section (expressed as percentage of all births).

	USA* (1978)	Dublin** (1984)
Abnormal labour	4.7	0.5
Repeat	4.7	1.1
Breech	1.8	0.5
Fetal distress	0.8	0.4
Others	3.2	1.7
	15.2	4.2

* *NIH Consensus Report*
** *National Maternity Hospital*

Caesarean rates were not a factor taken into account when the original decision was made to improve the quality of care extended to all women in labour in this hospital. Caesarean rates were simply not an issue 25 years ago, being much the same everywhere at about 5%. The low caesarean rates which have continued at this hospital through the intervening years must be seen as testimony to the fundamental truth: that efficient uterine action is the key to normal labour. Meanwhile, for the same reason, duration of exposure has been restricted and traumatic vaginal delivery, mainly in the form of rotational forceps, has been eliminated.[3]

Counting the cost

Given the lack of evidence that the massive increase in caesarean rates throughout much of the western world has resulted in any tangible benefits for infants, there are some pertinent questions to be asked. Does it really matter what the caesarean rate is in a particular hospital or community? At individual level, is it a matter of any great consequence that a woman's first baby is delivered by caesarean section, possibly under epidural anaesthesia with her husband present, if she is not likely to have more than two children in any event? For the obstetrician, who carries a dual responsibility, are there considerations of professional ethics insofar as the mother's welfare is concerned? Moreover, who created the medico-legal climate which is said to be a factor in many countries, and dominant in some? Finally, and perhaps most important of all, what are the repercussions of this radical change in practice on the Third World, from where so many graduates are trained in Western methods? Sooner or later these questions will have to be answered; they cannot be avoided indefinitely, as caesarean section rates continue to rise inexorably.

Figure 3. Correlation between caesarean and perinatal mortality rates

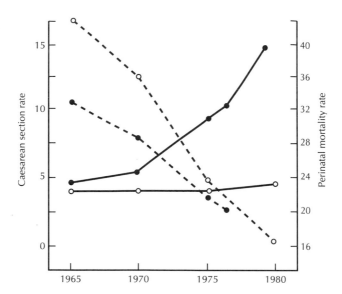

Caesarean section rates per 100 deliveries are represented by solid lines, and perinatal mortality rates per 100 deliveries by broken lines: in the USA according to Bottoms *et al.*[19] (circles), and in the National Maternity Hospital, Dublin[17] (crosses).

Summary

There has been an unwarranted increase in the caesarean birth rate in many countries in recent years. Most additional operations are performed on normal women – primigravidae with vertex presentation and single fetus – for the indication 'dystocia'. Inevitably, the more primary sections performed today, the more secondary sections will be necessary tomorrow. As effective uterine action is the key to normal labour, the central problem of dystocia can be solved by much simpler methods.

28: Cerebral Palsy

The influence of perinatal factors on subsequent neurological developments is a dominant concern in the wider context of reproductive medicine. Brain damage which could have been avoided may well be regarded as the ultimate failure in contemporary obstetric care. The traditional viewpoint – entrenched in the minds of many obstetricians, paediatricians and, indeed, the community at large – that cerebral palsy is, almost invariably, the result of asphyxia during labour, is seriously challenged by the results of the Dublin Trial, so called because it was conducted in this hospital.[13,20]

Hypoxia

Labour is a potential cause of asphyxia because blood flow through the placenta is always impeded by uterine activity: every uterine contraction reduces oxygen supply to the fetus. As labour progresses the cumulative effect may lead to a significant degree of hypoxia. This physiological process presents no problem to the well nourished fetus who enters labour with a normal placenta and sufficient reserve to adapt to labour of reasonable duration. On the other hand, the fetus whose reserve is already diminished before labour began is vulnerable to the stress of normal labour. To the fetus, the consequence is the same whether the natural action of the uterus is sufficient to dilate the cervix or inefficient uterine action is corrected with oxytocin.

Trauma

Trauma, in vertex presentation, is virtually confined to delivery by traction, particularly when preceded by rotation. In spontaneous delivery, trauma to the fetus, in vertex presentation, is a very rare event. Since the incidence of instrumental delivery falls sharply with augmentation of slow labour, oxytocin can reduce the risk of birth injury from this source.

Care of fetus during labour

Supervision of the fetus during labour is based on the simple premise that a healthy fetus and placenta, is competent to meet the stress of normal labour. To ensure early detection of a fetus which is already compromised by impaired placental function, but which has escaped recognition at the antenatal clinic, amniotomy is performed as soon as the diagnosis of labour is confirmed. Thereafter, supervision is by intermittent auscultation, performed for one full minute, at intervals of 15 minutes during the first stage and after every contraction during the second stage.

Research project

Because of the unresolved controversy concerning the respective values of continuous electronic monitoring and intermittent auscultation, a decision was made to compare the two methods in the context of the standardised practice established in this hospital. See Chapter 23. A prospective randomised trial was conducted over a period of two years. The results showed no difference in perinatal mortality rate. Neither was there a significant difference in Apgar scores, need for intubation or admission to Special Care Baby Unit. There was one significant difference: nine neonatal convulsions in the electronic group, compared with 21 in the control group. When these 30 infants were examined 12 months later, six showed evidence of brain damage; three were from the electronic group and three were from the control group.

At four years of age, reassessment of the 30 children who had survived neonatal convulsions, confirmed that six suffered from cerebral palsy: the same three from each group. A fourth child from the electronic group found to have cerebral palsy at four years had had transient neurological signs during the neonatal period. There were, in addition, 15 other cases of cerebral palsy who had had no abnormal signs during the neonatal period: eight were from the electronic group and seven were from the control group. At the end of four years, therefore, there were 22 cases of cerebral palsy: 12 from the electronic group and 10 from the control group. A finding of at least equal importance to the practice of obstetrics was, that only six of the total number of 22 cases of cerebral palsy at four years of age had shown any sign whatever of birth asphyxia.

Two firm conclusions are drawn from this classical study: first, that continuous electronic monitoring of the fetal heart during labour afforded no additional protection against cerebral palsy and, second, that cerebral palsy was not associated with previous birth asphyxia in most cases.

Summary

Routine use of electronic fetal heart monitors offer no advantage over standard clinical methods, either in terms of immediate survival or subsequent neurological development. In centres where sophisticated equipment may not be available, or affordable, this conclusion will be of particular interest. The additional finding, that almost three in four cases of cerebral palsy were not associated with birth asphyxia, has clear medico-legal implications.

Section II
Visual Records of Labour

Primigravid labour

Primigravid labour

There are fundamental differences between first and subsequent labour. These differences are so great that they warrant the statement that primigravidae and multigravidae behave as different biological species; proper management of labour rests on this premise.

- The causes of delay and risks of treatment are very different.
- The diagnosis of early labour is more difficult in the primigravida because the cervix must be effaced before dilatation begins.
- The duration of a first labour is longer because inefficient uterine action is commonplace and because the birth canal has not been stretched before.
- Inefficient uterine action is uncommon in parous women. Delay in multiparous labour is more often an expression of obstruction caused by a fetal complication, such as malformation or malpresentation, which can easily lead to rupture of the uterus.
- The primigravid uterus is immune to rupture.
- The multigravid uterus is prone to rupture.
- Oxytocin does not cause rupture of the primigravid uterus even in the presence of cephalopelvic disproportion.
- Oxytocin may cause rupture of the parous uterus even in normal labour.
- To ensure that this distinction is manifest at all times the Primigravid Labour Record is printed on yellow paper and the Multigravid Labour Record on blue paper.

GRAPH 1

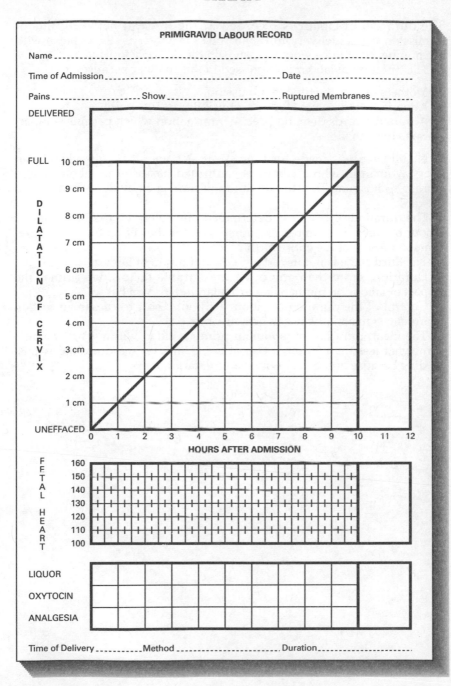

PRIMIGRAVID LABOUR RECORD

Name _____

Time of Admission _____ Date _____

Pains _____ Show _____ Ruptured Membranes _____

HOURS AFTER ADMISSION

Time of Delivery _____ Method _____ Duration _____

Duration of labour

The duration of labour is recorded as the interval between time of admission to the delivery unit and time of delivery. This equates with the number of hours a woman spends in the delivery unit.

The duration of labour is expressed in this manner because:

- Mothers decide the time of admission.
- Attendant staff assume their responsibility at this point.
- Accurate records demand precise information which permits comparisons to be made.

No allowance is made for time spent at home. It is self-evident that every woman in whom labour is confirmed has been in labour before coming to hospital. To estimate duration from such evidence is a shot in the dark.

The duration of labour is determined effectively by the first stage of labour because the number of hours taken for the cervix to dilate represents some 90% of the entire birth process.

The third stage is not included in the definition of labour.

Duration, more than any other measurable factor, determines the impact of labour on mothers in particular, but also on babies.

Control of the duration of labour without resort to caesarean section represents a major advance in obstetric practice.

The mean duration of labour in primigravidae without treatment is somewhat less than 6 hours. Use of the term 'average duration' is misleading because of the very wide natural variation.

GRAPH 2

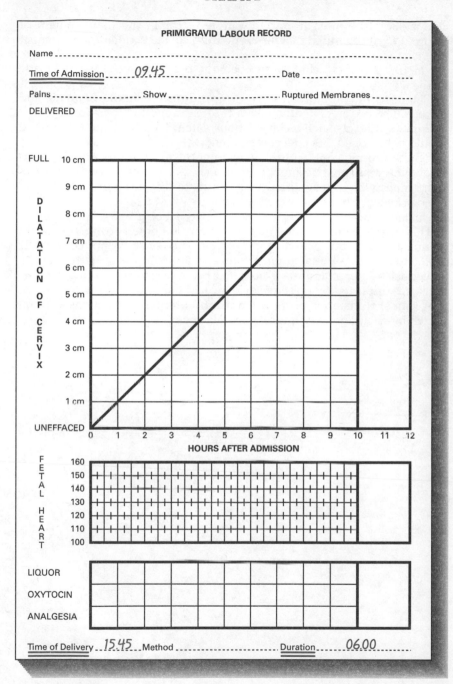

PRIMIGRAVID LABOUR RECORD

Name _____

Time of Admission _____ *09.45* _____ Date _____

Pains _____ Show _____ Ruptured Membranes _____

DELIVERED

FULL

DILATATION OF CERVIX

10 cm
9 cm
8 cm
7 cm
6 cm
5 cm
4 cm
3 cm
2 cm
1 cm

UNEFFACED

0   1   2   3   4   5   6   7   8   9   10   11   12

HOURS AFTER ADMISSION

FETAL HEART

160
150
140
130
120
110
100

LIQUOR

OXYTOCIN

ANALGESIA

Time of Delivery _____ *15.45* ____ Method _____ Duration _____ *06.00* _____

133

Diagnosis of labour

Diagnosis is the most important single factor in the management of labour. When the initial diagnosis is wrong, all subsequent management is likely to be wrong.

The first step is to confirm or reject the presumptive diagnosis made by the woman.

Diagnosis must be prospective. A firm decision should be made and placed on record not later than 2 hours after admission to hospital.

Equivocal terms such as false labour, latent labour or not established should not be used. Such terms represent evasion of responsibility.

Painful uterine contractions alone do not warrant a medical diagnosis of labour. Pains must be supported by a show or spontaneous rupture of membranes which provide invaluable aids to diagnosis in such circumstances, because both are objective in nature.

Dilatation of the cervix is the only proof of labour.

This graph records a woman who admits herself to hospital with painful uterine contractions and a show. The cervix is not completely effaced and, as a consequence, there is no dilatation of the cervix. Nevertheless, her diagnosis is accepted because painful uterine contractions are supported by objective evidence, in this case, a show.

A similar decision is made when painful uterine contractions are supported by spontaneous rupture of membranes.

GRAPH 3

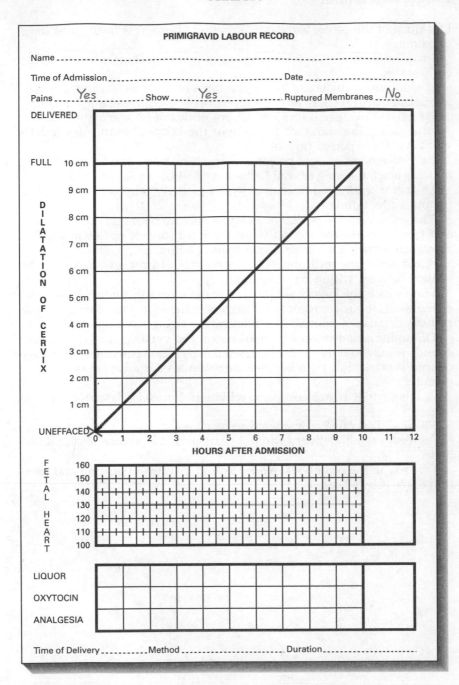

PRIMIGRAVID LABOUR RECORD

Name ....

Time of Admission .... Date ....

Pains ....*Yes*........ Show ....*Yes*........ Ruptured Membranes ...*No*....

DELIVERED

FULL   10 cm

DILATATION OF CERVIX
9 cm
8 cm
7 cm
6 cm
5 cm
4 cm
3 cm
2 cm
1 cm

UNEFFACED

0 1 2 3 4 5 6 7 8 9 10 11 12

HOURS AFTER ADMISSION

FETAL HEART
160
150
140
130
120
110
100

LIQUOR

OXYTOCIN

ANALGESIA

Time of Delivery .... Method .... Duration ....

135

Progress in labour

Dilatation of the cervix is the only criterion of progress in the first stage of labour.

Progress is monitored by vaginal examination at short intervals in the early stages.

A slow rate of dilatation in the first three hours is a clear indication of inefficient uterine action; rarely is cephalopelvic disproportion a factor.

At the end of three hours the pattern of dilatation is usually evident. At this point, the standard practice of the hospital is to inform each woman of the expected time of delivery.

Early diagnosis of slow progress is crucial to good management. Four hours is much too long to wait to discover that labour is abnormal.

Dilatation, expressed in centimetres, is plotted against time, expressed in hours, after admission.

The graph covers a period of 12 hours only: 10 hours for the first stage and two hours for the second stage; the third stage is not included. No provision is made for labour longer than 12 hours.

A diagonal line indicates the slowest rate of progress necessary to achieve delivery within this time limit.

Simplicity is the keynote in the design of this graph. Only the essential elements of labour are recorded. Progress in the first stage dominates the picture. Details not immediately relevant are rigorously excluded.

Dilatation at admission is marked on the vertical axis that corresponds with zero hour on the horizontal axis. A cervix that is completely effaced is marked at 1 cm because the external os is always open to this extent.

A labour that is not complete within 12 hours is classified as prolonged.

Prolonged labour is considered to be an indication for caesarean section unless vaginal delivery without trauma can be predicted within one hour.

Progress in the second stage is measured in terms of descent and rotation of the baby's head.

GRAPH 4

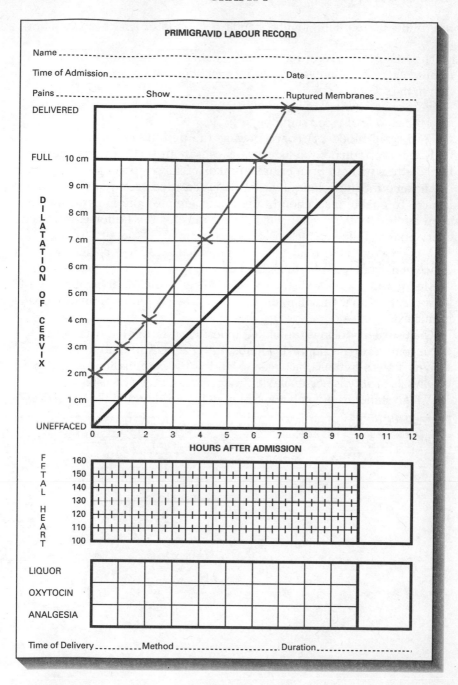

PRIMIGRAVID LABOUR RECORD

Name --

Time of Admission ----------------------------------- Date -----------------

Pains -------------------- Show --------------------------- Ruptured Membranes ----------

DELIVERED

FULL   10 cm

9 cm

8 cm

D
I
L
A
T
A
T
I
O
N

7 cm

6 cm

5 cm

O
F

4 cm

3 cm

C
E
R
V
I
X

2 cm

1 cm

UNEFFACED
    0   1   2   3   4   5   6   7   8   9   10   11   12

HOURS AFTER ADMISSION

F
E
T
A
L

160
150
140
130
120
110
100

H
E
A
R
T

LIQUOR

OXYTOCIN

ANALGESIA

Time of Delivery ---------- Method ------------------------- Duration ----------

137

Care of the fetus

Intermittent auscultation is the standard method of fetal heart monitoring.

The fetal heart is recorded by the woman's personal nurse for one full minute every 15 minutes during the first stage and after every contraction in the second stage.

Electronic fetal heart rate monitoring is used in selected cases only as an adjunct to fetal blood sampling.

Fetal scalp blood pH is accepted as the definitive test for hypoxia. Only in exceptional circumstances is caesarean section performed for fetal distress without prior examination of a fetal scalp sample.

The amount and colour of the liquor is accorded great potential significance. To enable inspection of the liquor, amniotomy is performed as soon as 'in labour' is confirmed. The nature of the liquor is recorded every hour as follows, C (clear), M (meconium) or N (none).

A good volume of clear liquor is regarded as almost conclusive evidence of normal feto-placental function.

Meconium raises a suspicion of fetal hypoxia, as does absence of liquor. Attention is drawn to the different grades of meconium described in the text.

The use of oxytocin is prohibited unless clear liquor has been seen.

Meconium or no liquor is an absolute bar to stimulation of uterine activity unless hypoxia has been excluded by examination of fetal pH. When this facility is not available, oxytocin should not be used.

A high standard of fetal monitoring in labour does not require sophisticated equipment.

GRAPH 5

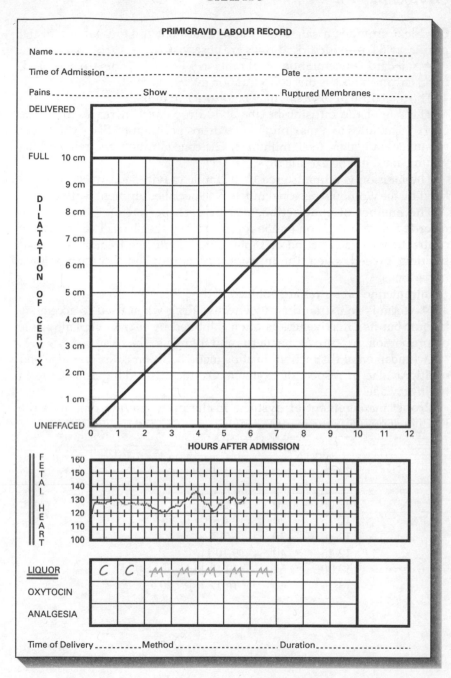

PRIMIGRAVID LABOUR RECORD

Name ....

Time of Admission .... Date ....

Pains .... Show .... Ruptured Membranes ....

DELIVERED

DILATATION OF CERVIX

FULL	10 cm
	9 cm
	8 cm
	7 cm
	6 cm
	5 cm
	4 cm
	3 cm
	2 cm
	1 cm
UNEFFACED	

0 1 2 3 4 5 6 7 8 9 10 11 12

HOURS AFTER ADMISSION

FETAL HEART

160 150 140 130 120 110 100

LIQUOR	C	C	M	M	M	M	M
OXYTOCIN							
ANALGESIA							

Time of Delivery .... Method .... Duration ....

139

Oxytocin

Oxytocin provides a safe and simple treatment of slow labour in the primigravida, provided rigid rules are observed.

A standard concentration of 10 units in 1 litre of 5% dextrose is used. In no circumstances is this concentration every changed.

The total dose of oxytocin may not exceed 10 units.

The rate of the infusion begins at 10 drops and increases 10 drops every 15 minutes to a maximum of 60 drops per minute. Sixty drops per minute is equivalent to 40 milliunits. The concentration, the rate and the volume must not be exceeded.

The infusion is administered by a simple gravity feed which is regulated by the woman's personal nurse. No special equipment is used.

The number of contractions during each period of 15 minutes is recorded in serial fashion on the reverse side of the chart. The aim is five contractions in each period of 15 minutes. Should the frequency of contractions exceed seven, the infusion rate is reduced to guard against hypertonus.

Intrauterine pressures are not recorded.

Oxytocin is an extraordinarily effective drug when used to accelerate labour, but its effectiveness is often inhibited by fear of cephalopelvic disproportion, rupture of the uterus and trauma to the baby.

A fundamental distinction must be made between primigravidae and multigravidae in respect of oxytocin. Oxytocin is a dangerous drug in multigravidae.

Proper management of dystocia in the primigravida demands the intelligent use of oxytocin.

Time	Rate	Contractions
12.00	10	1,2
12.15	20	3,4,5
12.30	30	6,7,8
12.45	40	9,10,11
13.00	50	12,13,14,15
13.15	60	16,17,18,19,20

GRAPH 6

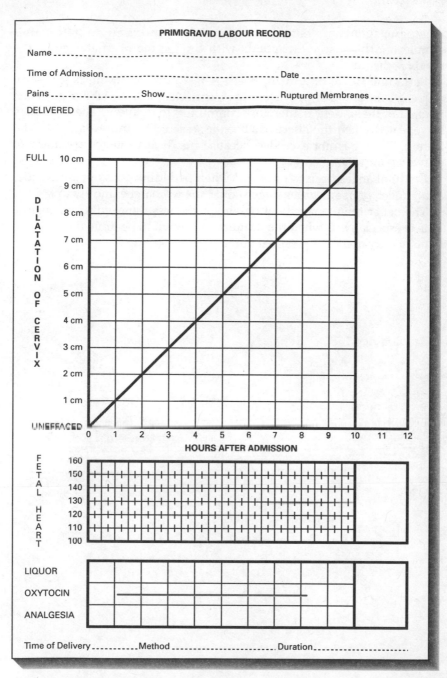

PRIMIGRAVID LABOUR RECORD

Name _____

Time of Admission _____ Date _____

Pains _____ Show _____ Ruptured Membranes _____

DELIVERED

FULL   10 cm

9 cm

D
I   8 cm
L
A   7 cm
T
A   6 cm
T
I   5 cm
O
N   4 cm

O   3 cm
F
2 cm
C
E   1 cm
R
V   UNEFFACED
I
X   0   1   2   3   4   5   6   7   8   9   10   11   12

HOURS AFTER ADMISSION

F   160
E   150
T   140
A   130
L   120
H   110
E   100
A
R
T

LIQUOR

OXYTOCIN

ANALGESIA

Time of Delivery _____ Method _____ Duration _____

Analgesia

Analgesic agents are entered in the space appropriate to hours after admission; this also corresponds with the degree of dilatation of the cervix at the time.

Pethidine is the only drug used. A test dose of 50 mg is given on request, subject to the provision that a firm diagnosis of labour has been made and the patient is therefore committed to delivery. The dose may be repeated when the effect has been assessed 30 minutes later. A total dose of 100 mg is not exceeded because the disadvantages are likely to outweigh the advantages.

Epidural anaesthesia is provided when pethidine does not afford adequate relief, or at an earlier stage should the woman be unduly upset.

The better the management of labour, the less the need for analgesia. This is especially so when the duration is known to be limited and every woman is assured of a personal nurse.

GRAPH 7

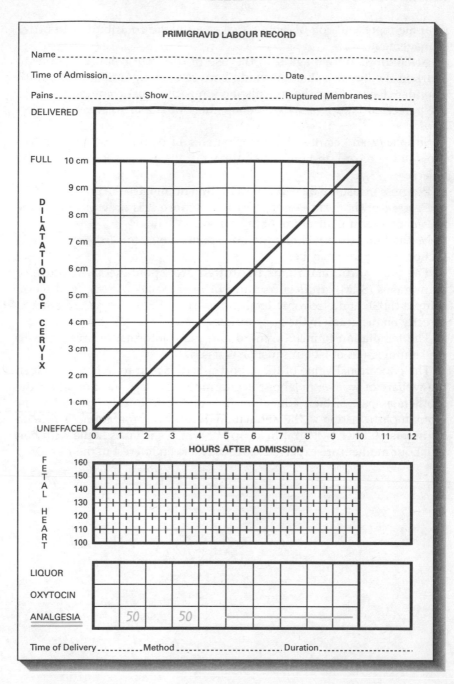

PRIMIGRAVID LABOUR RECORD

Name ....

Time of Admission .... Date ....

Pains .... Show .... Ruptured Membranes ....

DELIVERED

FULL

DILATATION OF CERVIX

10 cm
9 cm
8 cm
7 cm
6 cm
5 cm
4 cm
3 cm
2 cm
1 cm

UNEFFACED

0 1 2 3 4 5 6 7 8 9 10 11 12

HOURS AFTER ADMISSION

FETAL HEART

160
150
140
130
120
110
100

LIQUOR

OXYTOCIN

ANALGESIA   50   50

Time of Delivery .... Method .... Duration ....

143

Method of delivery and additional items

Graphic representation of labour makes a unique contribution to better management.

Attention is drawn again to the use of different coloured paper to sharpen the basic distinction made between primigravidae and multigravidae. Failure to make this distinction is the most common factor in the perceived failure of active management of labour to attain its objectives.

Simplicity and clarity of expression should be the most obvious features of the record. Instant visual impact of the essential elements is the objective.

Progress measured by cervical dilatation dominates the graph.

Descent of the head is not recorded because it is only of immediate relevance after full dilatation of the cervix.

Method of delivery is recorded as spontaneous, forceps or caesarean section, as the case may be.

The only additional items permitted are: spontaneous rupture of membranes (SRM), artificial rupture of membranes (ARM), fetal blood sample (FBS), and electronic fetal monitoring (EFM). These are entered directly on the graph in the appropriate place.

The temptation to include more and more information irrelevant to the central issues of labour must be resisted.

The educational value of these portraits of labour for all concerned in the welfare of women in labour is enormous; perhaps most of all for the mothers as part of their education for childbirth. In this hospital every woman participating in the antenatal educational programme is briefed to understand her partograph, a copy of which she takes home with her. In labour mothers are expected to display a keen interest in their graph.

GRAPH 8

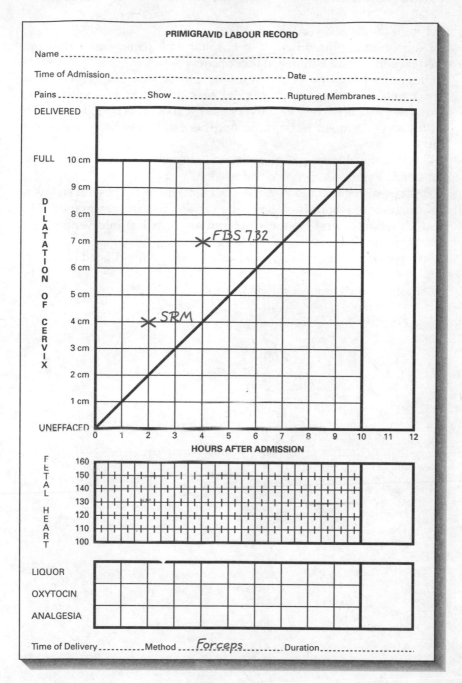

PRIMIGRAVID LABOUR RECORD

Name ....

Time of Admission .... Date ....

Pains .... Show .... Ruptured Membranes ....

DELIVERED

FULL

D I L A T A T I O N   O F   C E R V I X

FBS 7.32

SRM

UNEFFACED

HOURS AFTER ADMISSION

FETAL HEART

LIQUOR

OXYTOCIN

ANALGESIA

Time of Delivery .... Method .... *Forceps* .... Duration ....

145

Normal labour (1)

This is the profile of a very short labour.

The woman admitted herself to hospital with pains, show and ruptured membranes all within a matter of a few hours.

Diagnosis posed no problem as the cervix was discovered to be almost fully dilated on admission. She was surprised, and delighted to learn that she was so close to delivery after such a short period of time.

Progress continued to be rapid and her baby was born within the hour.

This case illustrates a poor correlation between time spent in labour at home and dilatation of cervix on admission.

This case also illustrates how misleading it can be to speak of an 'average' duration of labour because of the very wide natural variation. The mean duration of first labour – without any medical intervention – is somewhat less than 6 hours in this hospital.

Five per cent of all primigravidae are already fully dilated at admission.

Duration is the kernel of care in labour.

GRAPH 9

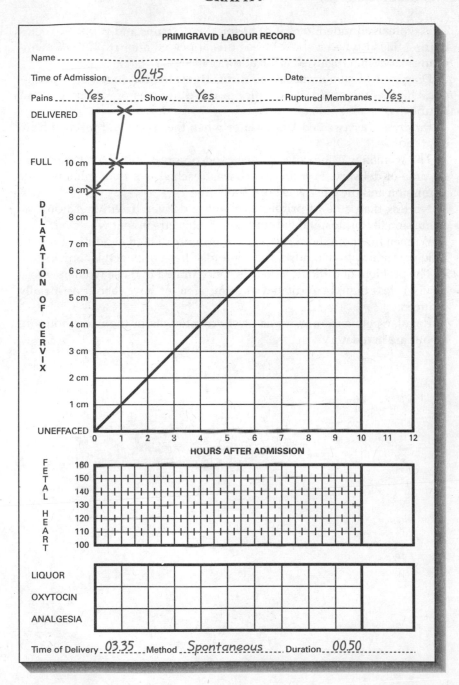

PRIMIGRAVID LABOUR RECORD

Name ....

Time of Admission .... _02.45_ .... Date ....

Pains ...._Yes_..... Show ...._Yes_.... Ruptured Membranes .._Yes_..

DELIVERED

FULL   10 cm

9 cm

8 cm

7 cm

6 cm

5 cm

4 cm

3 cm

2 cm

1 cm

UNEFFACED

DILATATION OF CERVIX

0 1 2 3 4 5 6 7 8 9 10 11 12

HOURS AFTER ADMISSION

FETAL HEART

160
150
140
130
120
110
100

LIQUOR

OXYTOCIN

ANALGESIA

Time of Delivery _03.35_ Method _Spontaneous_ Duration _00.50_

147

Normal labour (2)

This woman admitted herself to hospital with pains and ruptured membranes. She also had a show but as this appeared after rupture of membranes it was not regarded as an additional sign.

Diagnosis of labour caused no difficulty as the cervix was 3 cm dilated. This degree of dilatation places the diagnosis of labour beyond doubt.

Progress was assessed 1 hour later when the cervix had reached 5 cm dilatation.

The woman was informed of her good progress and given the expected time of delivery. Full dilatation was reached less than 4 hours after admission and the baby was born soon after.

No less than 40% of primigravidae are delivered within 4 hours of admission to this hospital without any medical treatment whatever.

Women in whom the cervix is 2 cm or more dilated at admission pose little problem with diagnosis and seldom suffer prolonged labour.

The problem of difficult labour is concentrated in those women whose cervix is less than 2 cm dilated at admission, or have labour artificially induced.

Regular pelvic examinations at short intervals in the early hours of labour are mandatory.

GRAPH 10

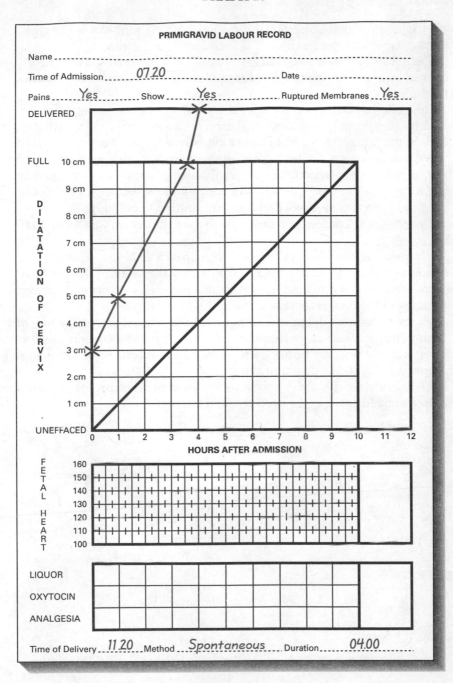

PRIMIGRAVID LABOUR RECORD

Name ....

Time of Admission .... *07.20* .... Date ....

Pains .... *Yes* .... Show .... *Yes* .... Ruptured Membranes *Yes* ......

DELIVERED

FULL   10 cm

DILATATION OF CERVIX

9 cm
8 cm
7 cm
6 cm
5 cm
4 cm
3 cm
2 cm
1 cm

UNEFFACED

0   1   2   3   4   5   6   7   8   9   10   11   12

HOURS AFTER ADMISSION

FETAL HEART

160
150
140
130
120
110
100

LIQUOR

OXYTOCIN

ANALGESIA

Time of Delivery .... *11.20* .... Method .... *Spontaneous* .... Duration .... *04.00* ....

149

Normal labour (3)

This woman admitted herself to hospital with painful uterine contractions only. There was no show. The membranes were intact.

Diagnosis of labour was confirmed because the cervix was completely effaced – there was objective evidence in support of painful uterine contractions.

Special attention is directed to the difference between effacement, which refers to the canal, and dilatation which refers to the external os and, in particular, the point of transition between these two events. Had this woman's cervix not been completely effaced her diagnosis of labour would not have been accepted in the absence of supportive evidence in the form of a show or spontaneous rupture of membranes. She would not have been retained and, therefore, committed to delivery.

Progress was confirmed 1 hour later when the cervix was 2 cm dilated.

Amniotomy was now performed to inspect the liquor. There was a free flow of clear (C) liquor, regarded as a virtual guarantee that feto-placental function is adequate to withstand the stress of normal labour. Prolapse of the cord is also excluded at this time.

Progress continued, but was sluggish, at the slowest acceptable rate of 1 cm per hour. Such cases demand frequent pelvic assessments at short intervals in the early hours of labour. Early detection of abnormal progress prevents the drift into abnormal labour.

Delivery was effected by forceps because of slow progress which ceased altogether when the head reached the perineum.

GRAPH 11

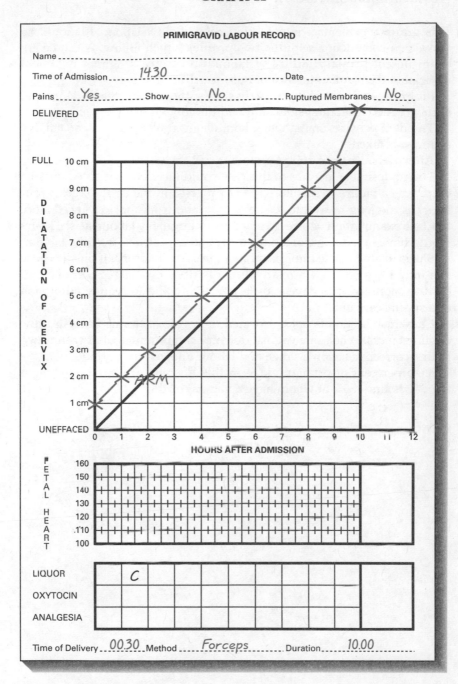

PRIMIGRAVID LABOUR RECORD

Name ....

Time of Admission .... *1430* .... Date ....

Pains .... *Yes* .... Show .... *No* .... Ruptured Membranes .... *No*

DELIVERED

FULL — 10 cm

DILATATION OF CERVIX

UNEFFACED

ARM

C

HOURS AFTER ADMISSION

FETAL HEART

LIQUOR

OXYTOCIN

ANALGESIA

Time of Delivery .... *00.30* .... Method .... *Forceps* .... Duration *10.00*

Abnormal labour: slow progress (1)

This graph represents a hypothetical case of slow labour. It should be viewed in conjunction with the two profiles which follow. All three are examples of primary failure of labour to progress, which is almost invariably the result of inefficient uterine action.

Progress was normal in the early stages, the cervix, dilating 1 cm per hour, reached 3 cm three hours after admission; all seemed well.

The next pelvic examination, 4 hours later, found the cervix 6 cm. No action was taken.

After 12 hours the cervix was close to full dilatation.

The undesirable features of this case could have been avoided. Firstly, there was a failure to monitor closely progress in the early stages – four hours is too long to wait to discover that labour has not advanced since the last examination. Corrective action to augment labour at six hours would have saved this woman from her bad experience of a long labour.

She is likely to have unpleasant memories of childbirth if only because she may have received a relatively large dose of analgesic drugs. Her baby is more likely to have a low Apgar score and to require admission to a special care unit.

Caesarean section is not performed on a rule of thumb basis in these circumstances. When safe vaginal delivery can be anticipated within two hours, corrective action is taken and labour allowed to continue.

Two per cent of primigravidae in this hospital are in labour longer than 12 hours – 80% of whom have a vaginal birth.

GRAPH 12

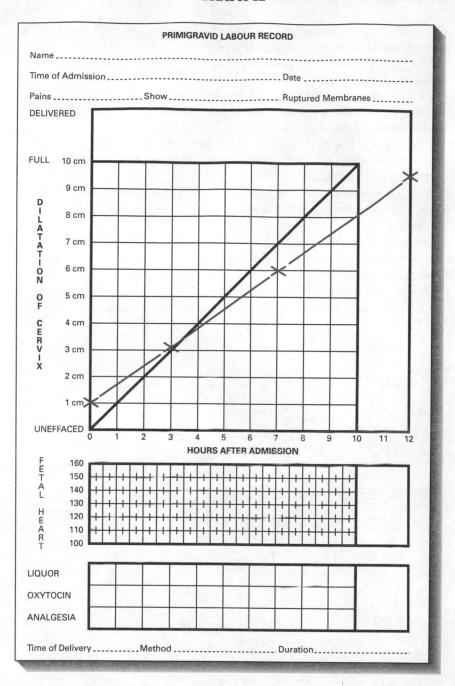

PRIMIGRAVID LABOUR RECORD

Name ....

Time of Admission .... Date ....

Pains .... Show .... Ruptured Membranes ....

Abnormal labour: slow progress (2)

This is the second example of a hypothetical case in which progress is even slower than in the previous instance.

Diagnosis of labour was not in question as the cervix was 2 cm dilated on admission.

Progress was negligible so that the cervix is little more than half dilated after 12 hours. In these circumstances it is clear that full dilatation will not be attained for many more hours.

There is also the likelihood of a difficult forceps delivery because the head may not descend and rotate, a situation fraught with serious risk of trauma to both mother and child.

This case exemplifies the passive 'wait and see' approach to childbirth, the most characteristic feature of which is prolonged duration of labour.

As in the previous case this woman is likely to have unhappy memories of her first experience of childbirth. As the only solution to her predicament is caesarean section she has also to contend with a section scar in the event of a future pregnancy.

Corrective action should have been taken at four hours.

GRAPH 13

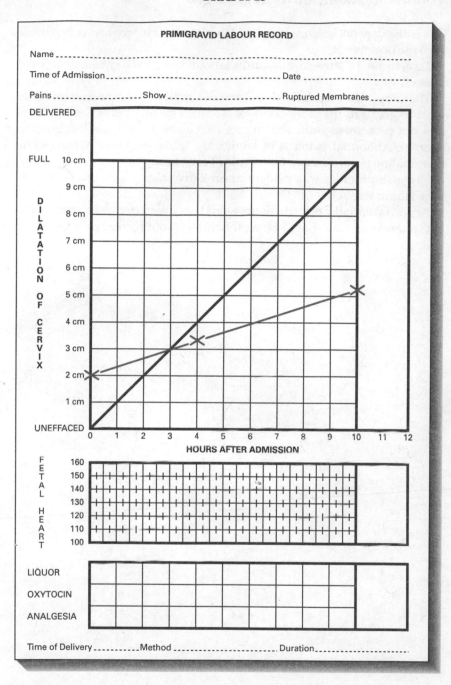

PRIMIGRAVID LABOUR RECORD

Name _____

Time of Admission _____ Date _____

Pains _____ Show _____ Ruptured Membranes _____

DELIVERED

FULL — 10 cm

9 cm

8 cm

7 cm

6 cm

5 cm

4 cm

3 cm

2 cm

1 cm

UNEFFACED

DILATATION OF CERVIX

0 1 2 3 4 5 6 7 8 9 10 11 12

HOURS AFTER ADMISSION

FETAL HEART

160
150
140
130
120
110
100

LIQUOR

OXYTOCIN

ANALGESIA

Time of Delivery _____ Method _____ Duration _____

Abnormal labour: slow progress (3)

This is the final notional case of slow labour in which progress is negligible from the beginning.

Twelve hours after admission in labour the cervix is less than 4 cm dilated.

The graph shows a failure to carry out regular pelvic assessments at short intervals in the early hours of labour. The first pelvic examination was not performed until four hours had elapsed – this is too long an interval. Abnormal patterns of labour are tacitly accepted when pelvic examination is performed at intervals of four hours.

Sluggish progress was evident at an early stage when the pattern of slow labour was set.

Action taken in the first few hours would have corrected the abnormality.

Caesarean section should be performed without further delay.

GRAPH 14

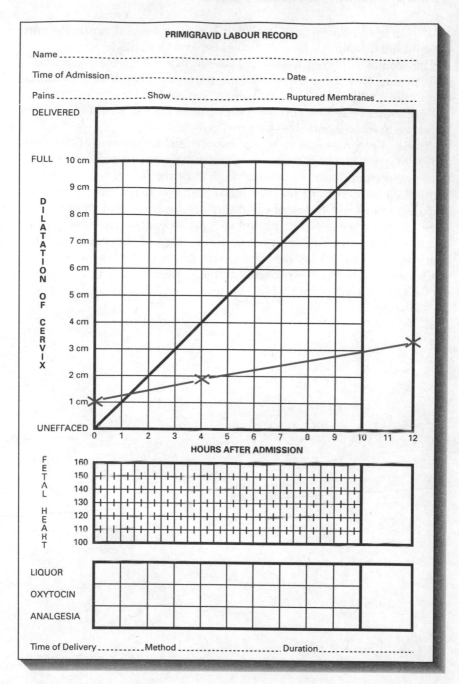

PRIMIGRAVID LABOUR RECORD

Name _____

Time of Admission _____ Date _____

Pains _____ Show _____ Ruptured Membranes _____

DELIVERED

FULL   10 cm
              9 cm
D   8 cm
I
L   7 cm
A
T   6 cm
A
T   5 cm
I
O   4 cm
N
              3 cm
O F
              2 cm
C
E   1 cm
R
V
I   UNEFFACED
X
              0   1   2   3   4   5   6   7   8   9   10 11 12

HOURS AFTER ADMISSION

F   160
E   150
T   140
A   130
L   120
            110
H   100
E
A
R
T

LIQUOR

OXYTOCIN

ANALGESIA

Time of Delivery _____ Method _____ Duration _____

157

Abnormal labour: secondary arrest (1)

This is an example of a case in which labour proceeded normally until close on full dilatation when no further progress was made.

The woman admitted herself because of painful uterine contractions and rupture of membranes, clear liquor was draining. Pelvic examination found a fully effaced cervix. Labour was confirmed.

Progress, assessed by repeated pelvic examination was normal until the cervix reached 8 cm when progress came to a halt.

Arrest of progress late in labour may be due to any one of the three causes of dystocia, but is more characteristic of cephalopelvic disproportion – or occipitoposterior position – than of inefficient uterine action. Nevertheless, inefficient uterine action remains the commonest cause and delay must not be ascribed to any other cause until oxytocin has been given for a restricted period of time to ensure efficient uterine action. This treatment identifies genuine cases of disproportion and bears no risk of rupture of the primigravid uterus or damage to the baby.

Oxytocin was given – progress immediately resumed and spontaneous delivery took place within 2 hours.

GRAPH 15

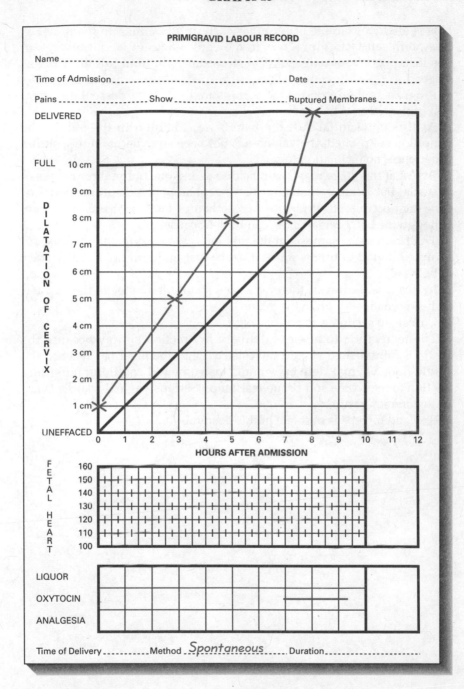

PRIMIGRAVID LABOUR RECORD

Name ....

Time of Admission .... Date ....

Pains .... Show .... Ruptured Membranes ....

Time of Delivery .... Method *Spontaneous* .... Duration ....

159

Abnormal labour: secondary arrest (2)

This is another example of secondary arrest. It is similar to the previous case, with satisfactory progress in the early stages of labour, except, in this instance, labour does not come to a standstill until full dilatation is reached.

Progress in the second stage is measured solely by descent and rotation of the head.

At this point in labour, the baby's head is high in the pelvis, the occiput is not rotated, the vagina has not been stretched and the mother experiences no inclination to push.

Arrest at this stage may again be due to any one of the three causes of dystocia, but is more characteristic of cephalopelvic disproportion – or persistent occipitoposterior position – than of inefficient uterine action, although the latter remains the commonest cause.

Treatment is the same as in the previous case – oxytocin is infused for a limited period of time with confidence that no harm can befall mother or baby.

In this case, however, there was no response to oxytocin, the unrotated head remained high in the pelvis.

Caesarean section was performed.

The temptation to attempt delivery by traction simply because the cervix is fully dilated should be resisted. Until the head has reached the pelvic floor vaginal delivery entails instrumental rotation and strong traction to overcome soft tissue resistance. Serious vaginal trauma is not an uncommon result.

Keilland forceps is obsolete in this hospital.

GRAPH 16

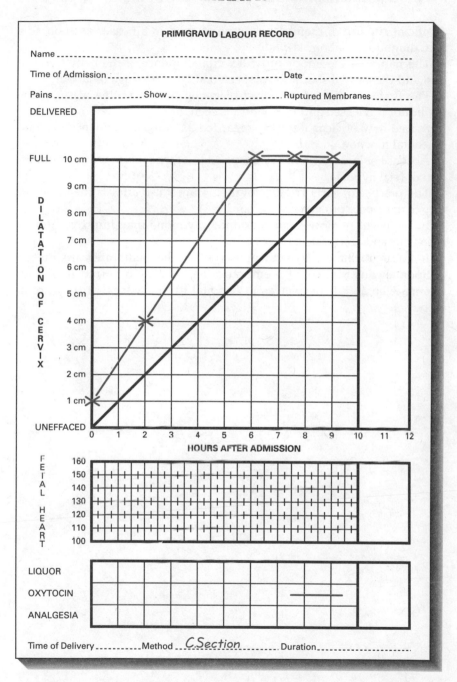

PRIMIGRAVID LABOUR RECORD

Name ....

Time of Admission .... Date ....

Pains .... Show .... Ruptured Membranes ....

DELIVERED

FULL — 10 cm

DILATATION OF CERVIX

9 cm
8 cm
7 cm
6 cm
5 cm
4 cm
3 cm
2 cm
1 cm

UNEFFACED

0 1 2 3 4 5 6 7 8 9 10 11 12

HOURS AFTER ADMISSION

FETAL HEART

160
150
140
130
120
110
100

LIQUOR

OXYTOCIN

ANALGESIA

Time of Delivery .... Method ... *C.Section* .... Duration ....

Method of treatment: artificial rupture of membranes

Artificial rupture of membranes is performed in all cases as soon as a firm diagnosis of labour is made.

The nature of the liquor provides vital evidence of the baby's condition and therefore it should be inspected at an early stage of labour.

The first suspicion of impaired placental function often arises when the liquor is released and meconium is seen.

A free flow of clear liquor is regarded as valuable evidence of good placental function.

Absence of liquor or a heavy suspension of meconium raises the question of fetal hypoxia.

The practice of early rupture of membranes also affords the opportunity to anticipate prolapse of the cord.

In the event of slow labour, amniotomy alone may improve uterine efficiency and accelerate progress.

In no circumstances is oxytocin used when the membranes are intact.

Spontaneous rupture of membranes has already occurred in 30% of women who admit themselves to hospital in the belief that they are in labour.

GRAPH 17

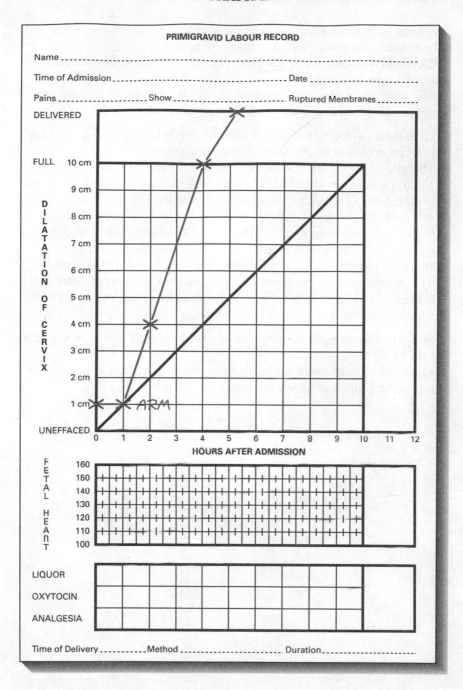

Method of treatment: oxytocin infusion (1)

One hour after artificial rupture of the membranes has been performed, pelvic examination is repeated to measure progress.

Oxytocin is started when dilatation has not increased by 1 cm, always provided clear liquor is seen.

The standard procedure applied in all circumstances and by every member of nursing and medical staff is as follows:

- 10 units of oxytocin in 1 litre of 5% dextrose solution is used. This concentration cannot be changed in any circumstances.
- The rate of the infusion starts at 10 drops per minute and increases by 10 drops at intervals of 15 minutes to a maximum of 60 drops per minute which is the equivalent of 40 milliunits. The concentration, the rate and the volume must not be exceeded, so it is not possible for a woman to receive more than 10 units of oxytocin, 1 litre of dextrose solution, or treatment lasting longer than six hours.
- A simple gravity feed is regulated by the woman's personal nurse.
- The number of contractions is recorded on the reverse side of the labour record. The number is not allowed to exceed seven in 15 minutes – hypertonus is thereby prevented.

Subject to these rigorous restrictions, fetal hypoxia is the only potential problem.

Oxytocin should *never* be used when there is evidence of impaired feto-placental function or fetal distress.

GRAPH 18

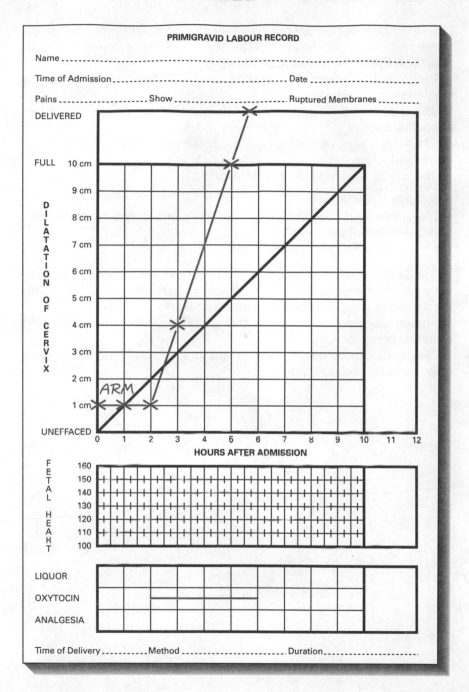

Method of treatment: oxytocin infusion (2)

This case illustrates the use of oxytocin in the second stage of labour.

Progress of labour was normal in the first stage, proceeding to full dilatation within a reasonable period of time.

Progress ceased early in the second stage – the head remained high in the pelvis, in an unrotated position.

The mother had no desire to push because there was no pressure on her pelvic floor.

The vagina was, of course, undilated; the woman was in Phase 1 of the second stage.

There were three options in treatment:

- Rotation and delivery.
- Caesarean section to avoid the possibility of a difficult rotation and delivery through an undilated vagina.
- Oxytocin for a limited period of time.

The latter option was taken, a standard oxytocin infusion was commenced, which resulted in descent and rotation of the head, thus avoiding a difficult and potentially dangerous delivery.

Should the head not reach the pelvic floor within 1 hour, caesarean section is performed.

Oxytocin can be an invaluable aid in the management of slow progress in the second stage.

GRAPH 19

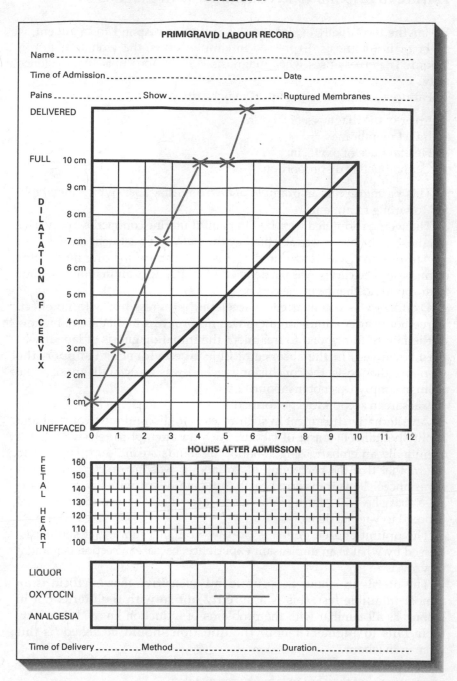

PRIMIGRAVID LABOUR RECORD

Name ....

Time of Admission .... Date ....

Pains .... Show .... Ruptured Membranes ....

DELIVERED

FULL   10 cm
        9 cm
        8 cm
D   7 cm
I   6 cm
L
A   5 cm
T
A   4 cm
T
I   3 cm
O
N   2 cm

O F   1 cm

C
E
R   UNEFFACED
V   0   1   2   3   4   5   6   7   8   9   10   11   12
I
X   HOURS AFTER ADMISSION

FETAL HEART   160
              150
              140
              130
              120
              110
              100

LIQUOR

OXYTOCIN

ANALGESIA

Time of Delivery .... Method .... Duration ....

Failure to respond to treatment: error in diagnosis

By far the most likely explanation of failure to respond to treatment, is an error in diagnosis. Expressed in simple terms, the woman is not in labour. The error arises when diagnosis is based on subjective evidence only.

Failure to respond to treatment may be due to:

- Error in the diagnosis of labour.
- Intact membranes.
- Hesitant use of oxytocin.
- Cephalopelvic disproportion.

This partograph is an example of a wrong diagnosis which inevitably led to wrong treatment.

The woman admitted herself with painful uterine contractions only. Her diagnosis of in labour was accepted by the staff, and treatment started.

Amniotomy was performed to inspect the liquor one hour after admission. The cervix was partially effaced. Pelvic examination one hour later found no change in the cervix.

Oxytocin was commenced to accelerate progress but with no effect. Three hours after admission there was no progress in dilatation. In view of the failure to respond to treatment the initial diagnosis of labour was then reviewed. In the absence of objective evidence to support the woman's diagnosis, the conclusion reached was error in diagnosis – the woman simply was not in labour.

Caesarean section was performed.

An alternative treatment in such cases is to discontinue treatment and await spontaneous onset of labour. Such an attempt to retrieve what is admittedly an embarrassing situation demands a candid explanation to the mother that the perception of 'in labour' was incorrect. In these circumstances she is transferred to an antenatal ward with a firm reassurance that she will return some hours later in spontaneous labour and proceed to vaginal delivery.

The option chosen depends on the woman's morale; if she is distressed by what is an unpleasant experience, caesarean section is mandatory.

The uterus in labour is so uniformly sensitive that oxytocin is an almost infallible test; this is assuredly not so with the uterus not in labour, as all familiar with the problems of induction know. When oxytocin fails to augment labour the question should be asked 'is this woman in labour?'

Ten per cent of women who admit themselves to hospital under the impression that they are in labour are mistaken.

GRAPH 20

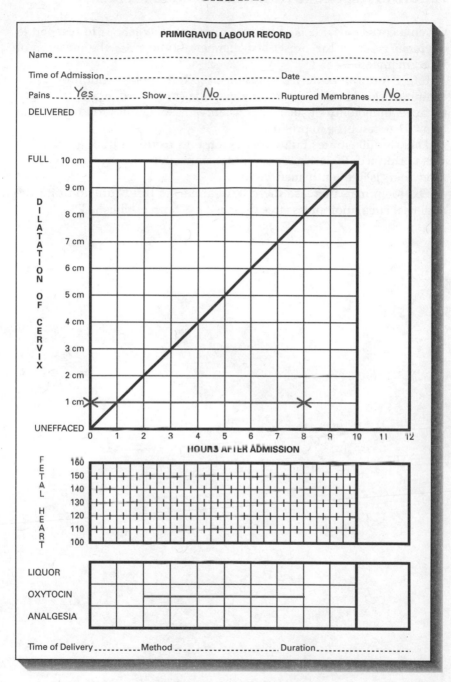

PRIMIGRAVID LABOUR RECORD

Name _____

Time of Admission _____ Date _____

Pains _____ *Yes* _____ Show _____ *No* _____ Ruptured Membranes ___ *No* ___

Time of Delivery _____ Method _____ Duration _____

Failure to respond to treatment: membranes intact

Given a correct diagnosis of labour, failure of slow labour to respond to oxytocin given in the prescribed manner should raise the question of intact membranes.

Intact forewaters may be present despite the observation of liquor draining. This possibility should always be considered at an early stage because amniotomy in such circumstances is sometimes followed by an immediate response in progress.

This case illustrates failure of response to oxytocin until amniotomy was performed. Experience shows that oxytocin in the presence of intact forewaters is frequently ineffective.

Oxytocin may increase the risk of amniotic fluid infusion into the maternal circulation unless free drainage has been established.

GRAPH 21

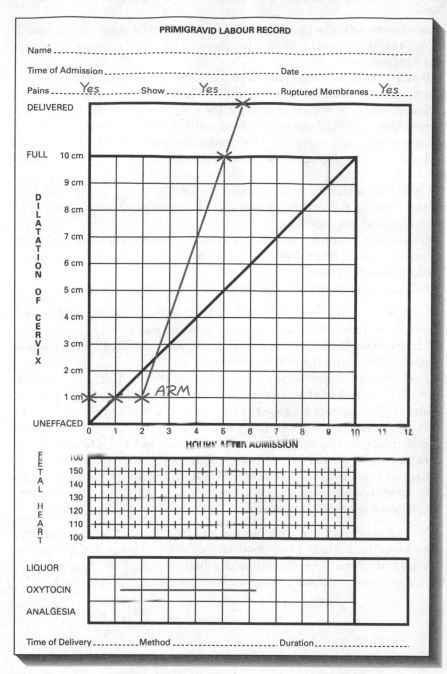

PRIMIGRAVID LABOUR RECORD

Name ....

Time of Admission .... Date ....

Pains .... Yes .... Show .... Yes .... Ruptured Membranes ... Yes

DELIVERED

FULL — 10 cm

DILATATION OF CERVIX
- 9 cm
- 8 cm
- 7 cm
- 6 cm
- 5 cm
- 4 cm
- 3 cm
- 2 cm
- 1 cm

ARM

UNEFFACED

0 1 2 3 4 5 6 7 8 9 10 11 12

HOURS AFTER ADMISSION

FETAL HEART
- 160
- 150
- 140
- 130
- 120
- 110
- 100

LIQUOR

OXYTOCIN

ANALGESIA

Time of Delivery .... Method .... Duration.......................

Failure to respond to treatment: hesitant use of oxytocin

This woman admitted herself with painful uterine contractions and a show. The cervix was completely effaced and her diagnosis of labour was confirmed.

Pelvic examination one hour later found the cervix 2 cm dilated – normal progress. Amniotomy was performed to inspect the liquor.

There was then failure to monitor the progress of labour in the early stages. Oxytocin was not commenced until five hours after amniotomy and the concentration was not increased at the prescribed rate.

Twelve hours after admission the cervix had reached only 5 cm dilatation.

Caesarean section was performed.

The pattern of dilatation of the cervix is not in any way suggestive of cephalopelvic disproportion.

Given that a woman is in labour and her membranes are ruptured, failure of slow labour to respond to treatment is almost certainly due to hesitant use of oxytocin.

Failure to use oxytocin in the prescribed manner may be due to:

- Failure to comprehend the difference between primigravidae and multigravidae in relation to rupture of the uterus.
- The die-hard belief that the merest possibility of cephalopelvic disproportion precludes the use of oxytocin.
- Lack of confidence between members of the medical and nursing staff. The sister in charge of the delivery unit is sure to begin with an ambivalent attitude because she has been educated to regard oxytocin as an extremely dangerous drug associated with rupture of the uterus and injury to the baby. Naturally she does not wish to accept the responsibility unless the most explicit assurances are given at the highest level. As this is seldom the case in practice, treatment comes to nought, while obstetricians wonder how it is that similar measures can prove successful elsewhere.

Mutual confidence between nurses and doctors, and indeed mothers, is an essential ingredient of good labour management but it must be carefully nurtured. The alternative is a high reported incidence of uterine hypertonus with fetal distress and cephalopelvic disproportion.

GRAPH 22

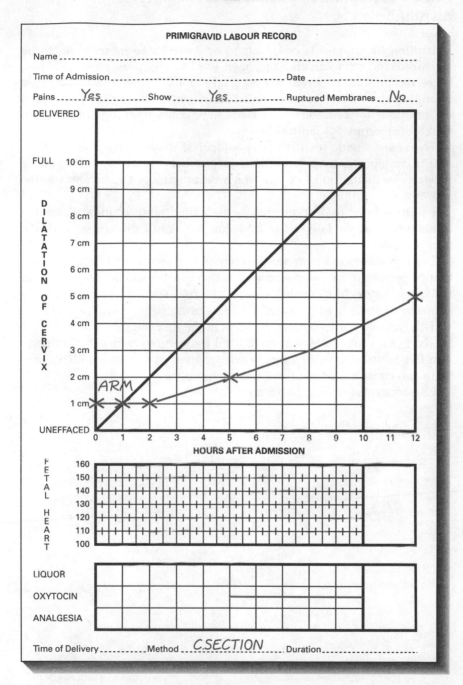

PRIMIGRAVID LABOUR RECORD

Name ....

Time of Admission .... Date ....

Pains .... *Yes* .... Show .... *Yes* .... Ruptured Membranes ... *No* ...

Time of Delivery .... Method .... *C.SECTION* .... Duration ....

173

Failure to respond to treatment: cephalopelvic disproportion

Assuming the diagnosis of labour to be correct, the membranes to be ruptured and oxytocin to have been used in the prescribed manner, there remain but two reasons why labour may continue to be slow: cephalopelvic disproportion and its clinical analogue, persistent occipitoposterior position. These two can be considered together because the clinical picture is identical.

The characteristic feature of cephalopelvic disproportion and persistent occipitoposterior position is failure of head to descend in spite of progressive dilatation of cervix which bears witness to efficient uterine action.

Failure of head to descend may be associated with secondary arrest in dilatation of cervix late in the first stage or at full dilatation, with the same outcome.

Even in these circumstances a diagnosis of cephalopelvic disproportion or persistent occipitoposterior position can seldom be made without the use of oxytocin to ensure efficient uterine action. X-ray pelvimetry contributed nothing to the solution of this essentially clinical problem.

This case illustrates secondary arrest in the first stage of labour treated by oxytocin. Progress was normal until the cervix reached 8 cm dilatation five hours after admission. When progress came to a standstill oxytocin was commenced but there was no response.

Caesarean section was performed.

GRAPH 23

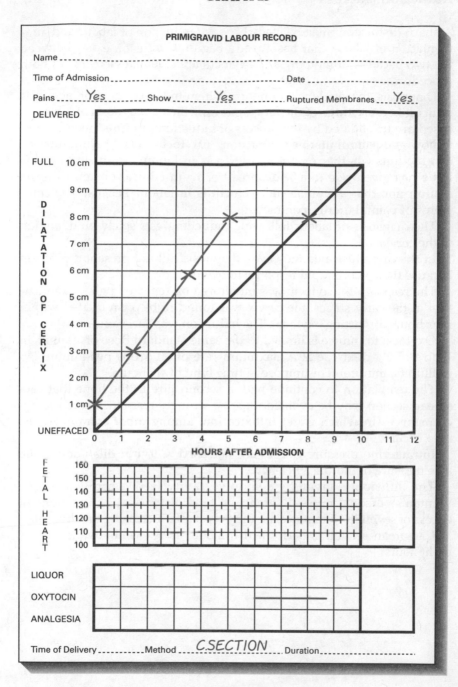

PRIMIGRAVID LABOUR RECORD

Name ....

Time of Admission .... Date ....

Pains .... *Yes* .... Show .... *Yes* .... Ruptured Membranes ..... *Yes*

DELIVERED

FULL   10 cm

DILATATION OF CERVIX

9 cm
8 cm
7 cm
6 cm
5 cm
4 cm
3 cm
2 cm
1 cm

UNEFFACED   0   1   2   3   4   5   6   7   8   9   10   11   12

HOURS AFTER ADMISSION

FETAL HEART

160
150
140
130
120
110
100

LIQUOR

OXYTOCIN

ANALGESIA

Time of Delivery .... Method .... *C.SECTION* .... Duration ....

175

Induction: success

A sharp distinction must be made between induction of labour and augmentation of labour that has already begun. Confusion exists between the two because amniotomy and oxytocin are essential elements of both procedures.

Diagnosis, the single most important item in the conduct of labour, is difficult because three of the four signs on which a diagnosis of labour is based are invalidated by the process of induction: ruptured membranes, a show and painful uterine contractions. Oxytocin causes painful uterine contractions whether or not a woman is in labour; confusion on this issue has given rise to a widespread error in clinical obstetrics – the assumption that a woman on oxytocin is in labour because she complains of painful uterine contractions.

The diagnosis of labour following induction rests solely on dilatation of the cervix.

In the case illustrated, however, diagnosis did not present a problem because there was a rapid response to oxytocin.

The response to oxytocin was monitored by repeated pelvic examination in the early stages; the cervix was found to be 3 cm dilated within four hours of starting oxytocin. The induction was successful.

Oxytocin to induce is limited to the same standard dose of 10 units in 1 litre of 5% dextrose at a maximum rate of 60 drops per minute (40 milliunits/minute). This imposes a time limit of six hours.

The temptation to continue with a second litre in the hope that caesarean section may be avoided must be strongly resisted. There are circumstances in which water intoxication, among other complications, may occur.

Intrauterine pressure gauges are not used. Cervical dilatation is the sole measure of uterine efficiency.

The infusion is given by a simply gravity feed controlled by the woman's personal nurse. Evidence of fetal distress, or contractions in excess of seven in 15 minutes are the only bar to increasing the drip rate.

Caesarean section is performed if labour is not well advanced after eight hours.

GRAPH 24

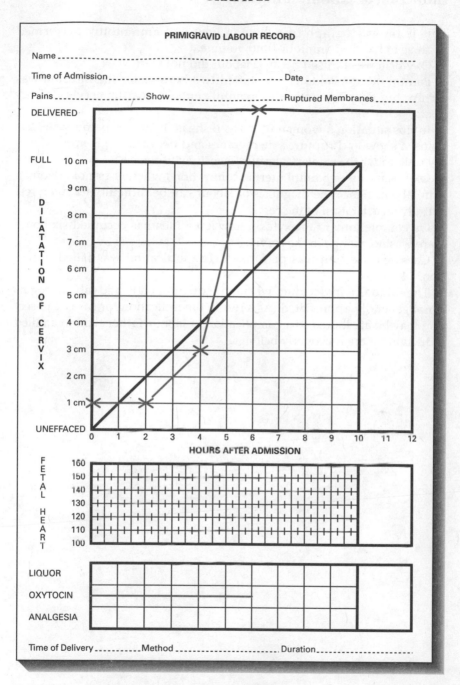

PRIMIGRAVID LABOUR RECORD

Name _____

Time of Admission _____ Date _____

Pains _____ Show _____ Ruptured Membranes _____

DELIVERED

FULL — 10 cm

DILATATION OF CERVIX

9 cm
8 cm
7 cm
6 cm
5 cm
4 cm
3 cm
2 cm
1 cm

UNEFFACED

0 1 2 3 4 5 6 7 8 9 10 11 12

HOURS AFTER ADMISSION

FETAL HEART

160
150
140
130
120
110
100

LIQUOR

OXYTOCIN

ANALGESIA

Time of Delivery _____ Method _____ Duration _____

Induction of labour: failure (1)

This is the partograph of a woman who had amniotomy performed because of reduced amniotic fluid volume.

Oxytocin was infused because labour did not start.

Painful uterine contractions started two hours after the infusion was set up, but despite continuing painful contractions the cervix did not dilate.

In this situation a woman reacts as if she is in labour, because she has pains, a show and ruptured membranes and because she is in the delivery unit under the same powerful suggestive influences.

Oxytocin causes painful uterine contractions whether or not a woman is in labour, hence the diagnosis of labour can be difficult and must rest entirely on dilatation of the cervix.

On completion of the oxytocin infusion which has occupied six hours there was no change in the cervix.

Caesarean section was performed. The indication was failed induction.

The difficulty in deciding when an induction ends and labour begins is not generally appreciated. As a result, the indication for caesarean section may be attributed to a complication of labour rather than to a failed induction where it properly belongs.

GRAPH 25

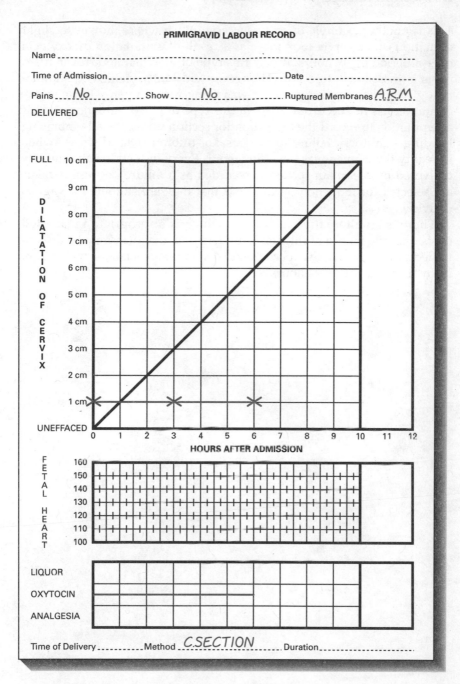

PRIMIGRAVID LABOUR RECORD

Name _____

Time of Admission _____ Date _____

Pains ___ *No* ___ Show ___ *No* ___ Ruptured Membranes *A.R.M*

DELIVERED

FULL — 10 cm

DILATATION OF CERVIX (9 cm, 8 cm, 7 cm, 6 cm, 5 cm, 4 cm, 3 cm, 2 cm, 1 cm)

UNEFFACED

HOURS AFTER ADMISSION (0 1 2 3 4 5 6 7 8 9 10 11 12)

FETAL HEART (160 150 140 130 120 110 100)

LIQUOR

OXYTOCIN

ANALGESIA

Time of Delivery _____ Method *C.SECTION* _____ Duration _____

179

Induction: failure (2)

This is another example of an unsuccessful case where, however, slight dilatation of the cervix took place as a result of stimulation by oxytocin over a period of six hours. It is in this type of case that an error in diagnosis is most likely to occur. The cervix reluctantly yielded to stimulation giving the impression that it was being forced open – but genuine dilatation has not occurred. Also, in this type of failed induction there is a temptation to record the indication for section under the all-embracing heading – dystocia, failure to progress, or dubious fetal distress –when in reality the woman was never in labour. Every induction subsequently delivered by caesarean section is recorded as a failure because patients are selected for induction on the basis that they are suitable for vaginal delivery.

There is an alternative to section, which is appropriate in selected cases once the nature of the case is understood; oxytocin may be discontinued in the reasonable expectation that spontaneous labour will start of its own accord within 24 hours.

GRAPH 26

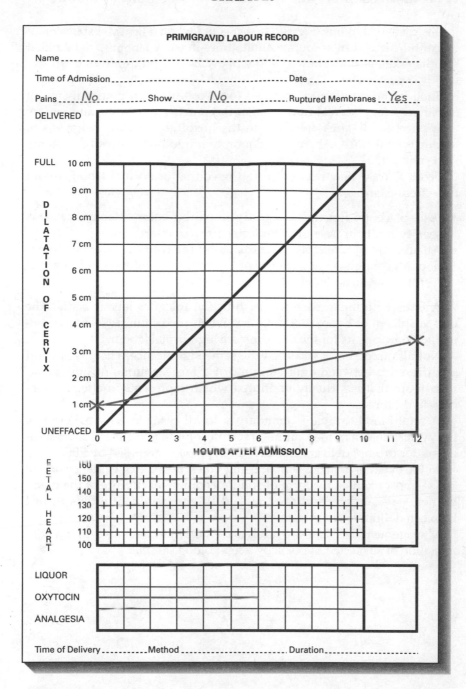

PRIMIGRAVID LABOUR RECORD

Name _____

Time of Admission _____ Date _____

Pains ___No___ Show ____No____ Ruptured Membranes ___Yes___

Time of Delivery _____ Method _____ Duration _____

Fetal distress: placental insufficiency/accident of labour

In this case fetal hypoxia was first suspected when a heavy suspension of meconium was seen at routine amniotomy in early labour. A fetal blood sample taken at once showed a low pH (7.2) and prompt caesarean section was performed.

Such is the significance attached to meconium as a potential sign of impaired feto–placental function that the practice of routine amniotomy is applied to all cases delivered in the hospital, once the diagnosis of labour is confirmed. Absence of liquor at amniotomy is treated with the same respect.

Fetal distress may occur during the course of normal labour under two circumstances:

- Feto–placental function is already impaired before labour begins as seen typically in cases of intrauterine growth retardation.
- An accident of labour such as prolapse of the cord or placental separation. Meconium is not a feature of the acute type of fetal hypoxia that results from an accident.

A fetus with impaired placental function tolerates labour badly. The first suspicion of hypoxia often arises when meconium is seen; meconium seldom appears for the first time during normal labour.

Not all meconium is accorded the same significance. There is a world of difference between light staining of a large volume of liquor and meconium that is virtually undiluted which represents in effect, severe oligohydramnios.

A fetal blood sample is mandatory in all cases in which there is a heavy suspension of meconium. Thick meconium is regarded as an indication for prompt delivery unless fetal hypoxia is excluded by FBS.

In the event of a blood sample being taken because of evidence of distress – most likely in the form of solid meconium at rupture of the membranes – a scalp electrode is attached to ensure a continuous record between definitive blood tests.

Management decisions are rarely based on EFM tracings without confirmation of suspected hypoxia by a fetal blood sample.

GRAPH 27

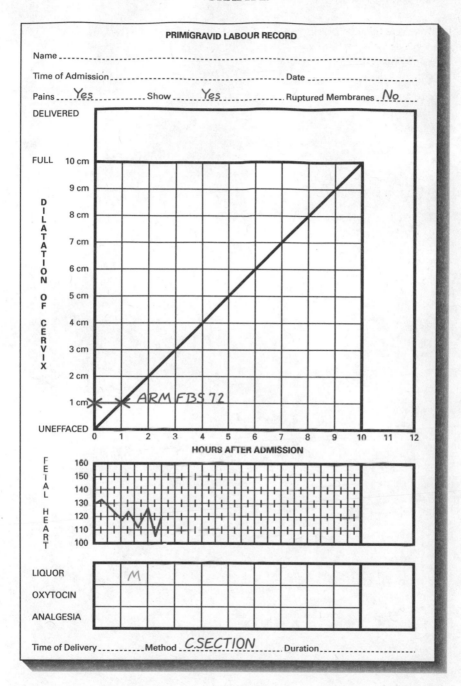

PRIMIGRAVID LABOUR RECORD

Name _____

Time of Admission _____ Date _____

Pains ___ *Yes* _____ Show _____ *Yes* _____ Ruptured Membranes __ *No* ___

DELIVERED

DILATATION OF CERVIX

FULL — 10 cm

9 cm

8 cm

7 cm

6 cm

5 cm

4 cm

3 cm

2 cm

1 cm ✗ — ✗ *ARM FBS 72*

UNEFFACED

0 1 2 3 4 5 6 7 8 9 10 11 12

HOURS AFTER ADMISSION

FETAL HEART

160
150
140
130
120
110
100

LIQUOR   *M*

OXYTOCIN

ANALGESIA

Time of Delivery _____ Method ___ *C.SECTION* _____ Duration _____

183

Multigravid labour

Multigravid labour

From the standpoint of labour the multigravid or parous woman might as well belong to a different biological species. Hence the labour record is printed on a different colour paper. Significantly, the sole difference in content is that the word 'Oxytocin' is omitted. Lack of appreciation of the reasons for these distinctions leads to the most prevalent of all obstetric errors: the practice of extrapolating from a first to a second labour. This results in much unnecessary intervention and iatrogenic disease. There is no basis for comparison as the events are completely unrelated. The salient features of multigravid labour may be summarised thus:

- The duration and consequent stress involved bear no comparison with first labour because the parous woman rarely suffers from inefficient uterine action and because her genital tract has been stretched before.
- In the event of slow progress therefore another explanation should be sought, the most likely being that she is not in labour.
- Failure to advance in a parous woman who is in labour is often a manifestation of obstruction arising from a fetal cause. This can be easily overlooked with disastrous consequences because the capacity of the pelvis is taken for granted.
- The common causes of obstruction are brow presentation and hydrocephalus.
- The parous uterus is prone to rupture and this may occur even in the course of normal labour.

Oxytocin should be used to stimulate the parous uterus only after most serious consideration and on a strictly individual basis. The diagnosis of labour should be reviewed and the causes of obstruction carefully excluded beforehand.

Epidural anaesthesia has very little application in the parous woman because one in two can expect to be delivered within two hours. In the event of slow progress, epidural anaesthesia is potentially dangerous because it permits labour to continue while suppressing evidence of impending rupture. The combination of oxytocin with epidural is particularly dangerous in this regard. Commitment to epidural anaesthesia in a parous woman is based on the false premise that all labours are the same.

GRAPH 28

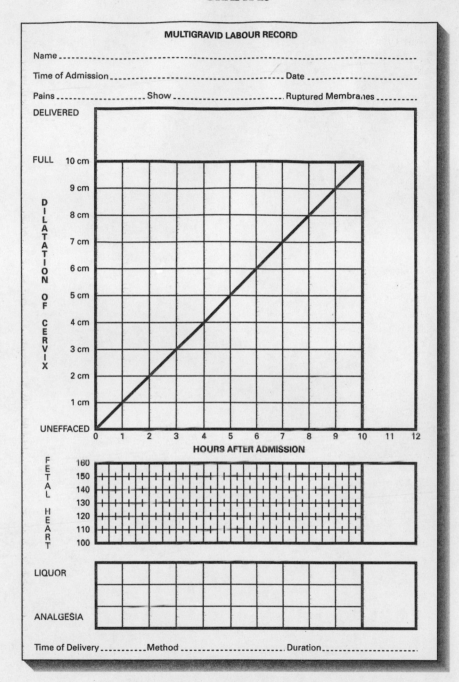

MULTIGRAVID LABOUR RECORD

Name ....

Time of Admission .... Date ....

Pains .... Show .... Ruptured Membranes ....

DELIVERED

FULL 10 cm

9 cm

8 cm

DILATATION OF CERVIX

7 cm

6 cm

5 cm

4 cm

3 cm

2 cm

1 cm

UNEFFACED

0 1 2 3 4 5 6 7 8 9 10 11 12

HOURS AFTER ADMISSION

FETAL HEART

160
150
140
130
120
110
100

LIQUOR

ANALGESIA

Time of Delivery .... Method .... Duration ....

187

SECTION III
Clinical Data

Comparative figures for 25 years

This table requires little in the way of explanation. As the general principle which underlies the practice of this hospital is to achieve the best results with the least interference, attention is directed to the following items:

Mortality rate

Perinatal mortality still represents the best objective measure of standards of practice in terms of the child. Notice is drawn to the exceptional number of post-mortem examinations performed. This has special relevance to trauma: death is all too easily attributed to hypoxia without post-mortem examination.

Caesarean section

In terms of the mother caesarean section rates serve the same function. The incidence of caesarean section has increased in recent years and has plateaued to 8%. These figures stand in sharp contrast with levels of 15 or 20% in similar institutions elsewhere.

Induction

The incidence of induction increased to 36% in 1970. Thereafter there was an abrupt decline when a selective, rather than statistical, approach to poorly defined risk factors, mainly pre-eclampsia and post-maturity, was adopted.

Forceps

For ease of comparison with other centres, the incidence of forceps deliveries is expressed here as a percentage of total births, whereas in practice some 90% of forceps deliveries were performed in primigravidae. With the introduction of active management of labour as standard procedure, the incidence of forceps deliveries declined to approximately 6%. Rotation forceps are not available in the hospital.

Table 1 Comparative figures for 25 years at the National Maternity Hospital.

Year	1965	1970	1975	1980	1985	1990	1992
Babies born	5063	6255	7430	8849	7482	6039	6256
Perinatal deaths	185	180	157	126	98	64	57
Necropsies	181	180	157	122	97	58	53
Mortality rate	36.5	28.3	21.1	14.2	13.1	10.6	9.0
Caesarean section (%)	4.2	4.2	4.1	4.9	5.1	8.5	8.5
Induction (%)	28.5	36.0	14.7	13.4	6.7	14.1	11.6
Forceps (%)	12.2	7.7	11.0	6.5	5.4	6.5	5.7

Analysis of hospital population

A progressive reduction in the perinatal mortality rate of some 66% over these 25 years was associated with notable changes in the background of the population served. There can be little doubt that these changes contributed more to the improvement in this respect than any advance in medical science. The chief items are listed in *Table 2*.

Maternal age

Maternal age has an important bearing on perinatal mortality. There has been a steady decline in incidence of mothers aged 40 or more with a corresponding increase in those aged less than 20.

Parity

A similar change was evident in the pattern of fertility. The percentage of grande multiparae declined by more than one half – from 23 to 7 with a corresponding increase in proportion of first births.

Birth weight

The incidence of low birth weight has remained low, consistently less than 10%. The progressive decline, to 3% in the 1980s, has not continued.

Table 2 Analysis of hospital population* at the National Maternity Hospital.

Year	1965	1970	1975	1980	1985	1990
Maternal Age						
<20	3	6	8	6	8	9
20–29	50	58	61	60	55	47
30–39	39	31	27	32	35	41
40+	8	5	4	2	2	3
Parity						
1	26	33	38	35	35	36
2,3,4	51	51	52	55	57	57
5+	23	16	10	10	8	7
Birthweight						
2.5 kg or less	7	6	4	3	3	5

* *Expressed to the nearest per cent.*

Clinical circumstances of perinatal deaths

This table places perinatal deaths in the clinical context in which they occurred. There were considerable improvements under all headings except one: died before labour.

By way of contrast the reductions elsewhere are the more striking because they occurred against the background of an increase of more than 50% in total births.

Dead when referred

The virtual elimination of this category of death reflects the trend to combined antenatal care and eventual hospital delivery, which took place at national level during these years; this item accounts for a reduction of 4 per 1,000 in the overall perinatal mortality rate.

Died before labour

This category includes late fetal deaths which occurred before the onset of labour. Most were unexplained but intrauterine growth retardation was a common finding. Improvement under this heading accounts for 4 per 1,000 in the perinatal mortality rate.

Died in labour ward

Apropos the management of labour, which is the subject of this manual, the improvement here represents a reduction of 2 per 1,000 in the perinatal mortality rate.

Neonatal deaths

This category accounts for a reduction of 8 per 1000 in the perinatal mortality rate, which should be considered in the light of the decline in the incidence of low birth weight referred to in *Table 2*.

Congenital malformations

The reduction under this heading, which accounts for 7 per 1000 in the perinatal mortality rate, appears to be the result of spontaneous improvement in the natural history of reproduction in the community.

Table 3 Clinical circumstances of perinatal deaths at the National Maternity Hospital.

Year	1965	1970	1975	1980	1985	1990
Total births	5063	6255	7430	8849	7482	6039
Dead when referred	22	16	8	4	0	1
Died before labour	43	56	70	57	41	26
Died in labour ward	16	24	8	10	11	7
Neonatal deaths	47	40	38	20	10	8
Congenital malformations	57	44	33	35	36	22
Total deaths	185	180	157	126	98	64

Rupture of uterus

This is the ultimate expression of serious injury to the mother. There was no case of rupture of uterus in more than 65,000 consecutive primigravidae delivered during a period of 25 years – despite the fact that oxytocin was used in some 25,000 to ensure efficient uterine action during labour – and without regard to the possibility of cephalopelvic disproportion.

Dehiscence of a caesarean section scar accounted for 64 of 92 cases of rupture of uterus in multigravidae.

The confidence necessary to use oxytocin effectively derives ultimately from the information contained in this and *Table* 5.

Table 4 Rupture of uterus at the National Maternity Hospital.

Year	1965	1970	1975	1976	1977	1978	1979	1980	1981	1982
Cases	4	8	4	5	4	5	6	3	5	3
Primigravidae	0	0	0	0	0	0	0	0	0	0

Year	1983	1984	1985	1986	1987	1988	1989	1990	TOTAL
Cases	2	2	1	2	2	1	0	2	92
Primigravidae	0	0	0	0	0	0	0	0	0

Traumatic intracranial haemorrhage in firstborn infants

This is the ultimate expression of serious injury to the child.

There were 45 cases of traumatic intracranial haemorrhage in firstborn infants: 22 cephalic and 23 breech presentations. All but two of the 22 cases of traumatic intracranial haemorrhage in firstborn infants with cephalic presentations were delivered with forceps.

Traumatic intracranial haemorrhage occurred twice in association with spontaneous vertex delivery in almost 65,000 firstborn infants and in neither case was oxytocin used.

This should be read in conjunction with *Table 4*.

Table 5 Traumatic intracranial haemorrhage in firstborn infants at the National Maternity Hospital.

Year	1965	1970	1975	1980	1985	1990	TOTAL
Births	1327	2054	2778	3106	2619	2114	64217
TICH	6	2	4	0	6	1	45
Breech	2	1	3	0	3	1	23
Vertex	4	1	1	0	2	0	22
Forceps	4	1	1	0	1	0	20

Cerebral dysfunction in mature infants

Permanent brain damage which could have been avoided may well be regarded as the ultimate failure in obstetric practice. So that these may be known and kept under surveillance, all cases of cerebral dysfunction identified in the course of routine examination for this purpose by our neonatologists, are placed on record.

Cerebral dysfunction is defined as a state of abnormal muscle tone or altered primitive reflexes which occurs in term infants who weigh 2,500 g. Preterm infants born before 37 completed weeks and infants of low birth weight are specifically excluded.

Hypoxia is clearly the most important factor in this regard, and typically this was the penultimate stage in a process which had existed before labour began: placental insufficiency in other words. Accidents of labour cover prolapse of cord and abruption of placenta. Among the cases of trauma there were six forceps and three breech deliveries. Other causes include drugs, infections and metabolic disorders.

Table 6 Cerebral dysfunction in mature infants at the National Maternity Hospital.

Year	1970	1975	1980	1985	1990	TOTAL
Babies born	6255	7430	8849	7482	6039	158342
Cerebral dysfunction	17	25	29	23	15	375
Hypoxia	12	17	23	18	11	283
Accident of labour	3	5	1	2	0	30
Trauma	0	0	1	1	0	12
Other causes	2	3	4	2	4	50

Diagnosis of labour

This table lists the evidence with which 1,000 consecutive primigravidae presented at the delivery unit of this hospital in the belief that labour had started.

Clearly some 10% were mistaken, because they failed to pass the initial test of painful uterine contractions. A very high proportion of those who passed this test had the additional evidence of a 'show' or spontaneous rupture of membranes. Notice was taken of a 'show' only when this appeared before the membranes ruptured.

Some with painful uterine contractions had neither of these two signs, in which case the crucial decision as to whether or not to retain was based entirely on complete effacement of the cervix.

Table 7 Diagnosis of labour at the National Maternity Hospital in 1000 consecutive primigravidae.

Pains	890
'Show'	586
Spontaneous rupture of membranes	269

Duration of labour in primigravidae

Duration of labour is synonymous with the time spent in the delivery unit of this hospital before the baby is born: all cases are included, whether or not a state of labour existed – a point of special significance in induction.

The mean duration of labour in primigravidae, without treatment, is somewhat less than 6 hours.

The composite figures given opposite are, like those in the next table, based on two series, each of 1,000 consecutive primigravidae, 5 years apart; treated cases are included.

Table 8 Duration of labour in primigravidae at the National Maternity Hospital.

Hours	%
< 2	12
2–4	26
4–6	28
6–8	20
8–10	9
10–12	3
12+	2
	100

Dilatation at admission in primigravidae

Effacement of the cervix refers to the length of the canal, from above downwards.

Dilatation of the cervix refers to the external os only, when effacement is complete.

The cervix is not effaced in some 7% and is already fully dilated in some 5% of primigravidae admitted to this hospital in labour. These two extremes do not relate well with the time spent in labour at home.

Many authors adopt the simple device of excluding those cases at the lower levels of dilatation and in doing so exclude the problem cases, both in diagnosis and treatment.

The multigravid cervix is an extremely different organ.

Table 9 Dilatation at admission in primigravidae at the National Maternity Hospital.

	%
Not effaced	7
Effaced	54
2, 3 cm	24
4, 5 cm	4
6, 7 cm	3
8, 9 cm	3
Full dilatation	5
	100

Obstetrical norms in primigravidae

A paradoxical feature of contemporary practice is a steady increase, almost everywhere, in the rate of medical or, more important, surgical intervention, despite a remarkable improvement in general health and a precipitous fall in perinatal mortality. There is indeed, a widespread tendency to attribute these improved results to this very intervention. *Table 1* shows how false this assumption can be; this table suggests that obstetricians might be better advised simply to hold the line as results continue to improve. Certainly, above anything else, iatrogenic disease – whether physical or emotional – must be avoided.

In conclusion, therefore, and based largely on experience recounted here, certain norms have been adopted to ensure that the rising tide of intervention is kept in check. The figures for multigravidae are lower – generally much lower – under each heading.

Table 10 Obstetrical norms in primigravidae at the National Maternity Hospital.

	%
Caesarean section	5
Induction	10
Forceps	10
Acceleration	45
Epidural	15

References

[1] O'Driscoll, K., Jackson, R.J.A., and Gallagher, J.T. (1969) Prevention of prolonged labour. *British Medical Journal*, **ii**: 477–480.

[2] O'Driscoll, K., Stronge, J.M., and Minogue, M. (1973) Active management of labour. *British Medical Journal*, **iii**: 135–137.

[3] O'Driscoll, K., Foley, M., and MacDonald, D. (1984) Active management of labor as an alternative to caesarean section for dystocia. *Obstetrics and Gynaecology*, **63**: 485–490.

[4] O'Driscoll, K. and Stronge, J.M. (1975) The active management of labour. *Clinics in Obstetrics and Gynaecology*, **2**: 3–17.

[5] Boylan, P., and O'Driscoll, K. (1983) Improvement in perinatal mortality rate attributed to spontaneous preterm labor without use of tocolytic agents. *American Journal of Obstetrics and Gynaecology*, **145**: 781–783.

[6] Boylan, P. (1976) Oxytocin and neonatal jaundice. *British Medical Journal*, **ii**: 564–565.

[7] O'Driscoll, K., Jackson, R.J.A., and Gallagher, J.T. (1970) Active management of labour and cephalopelvic disproportion. *British Journal of Obstetrics and Gynaecology*, **77**: 385–389.

[8] O'Driscoll, K. and Stronge, J.M. (1975) Active management of labour and occipito-posterior position. *Australian and New Zealand Journal of Obstetrics and Gynaecology*, **15**: 1–4.

[9] Daw, E., (1973) *Journal of Obstetrics and Gynaecology of the British Commonwealth*, **80**: 734

[10] O'Driscoll, K., Meager, D., MacDonald, D., and Geoghegan, F. (1981) Traumatic intracranial haemorrhage in firstborn infants and delivery with obstetric forceps. *British Journal of Obstetrics and Gynaecology*, **88**: 577–581.

[11] O'Driscoll, K. (1975) An obstetrician's view of pain. *British Journal of Anaesthesia*, **47**: 1053–1059.

[12] O'Driscoll, K., Coughlan, M., Fenton, V., and Skelly, M. (1977) Active management of labour: care of the fetus. *British Medical Journal*, **ii**: 1451–1453.

[13] MacDonald, D., Grant, A., Sheridan-Pereira, M., Boylan, P, and Chalmers, I. (1985) The Dublin randomized controlled trial of intrapartum fetal heart rate monitoring. *American Journal of Obstetrics and Gynaecology*, **152**: 524–539.

[14] Garcia, J., Curry, M., MacDonald, D., Elbourne, D. and Grant, A. (1985) Mothers' views of continuous electronic fetal heart monitoring and intermittent auscultation in a randomized controlled trial. *Birth*, **12**: 79–85.

[15] O'Driscoll, K., Carroll, C.J., and Coughlan, M. (1975) Selective induction of labour. *British Medical Journal*, **iv**: 727–729.

[16] O'Driscoll, K. (1972) Impact of active management on delivery unit practice. *Proceedings of the Royal Society of Medicine*, **65**: 697–698.

[17] O'Driscoll, K., and Foley, M. (1983) Correlation of decrease in perinatal mortality and increase in caesarean section rates. *Obstetrics and Gynaecology*, **61**: 1–5.

[18] US Department of Health and Human Services, Public Health Service, National Institutes of Health. Consensus Development Report: *Caesarean Childbirth*. No. 82-2067, October 1981.

[19] Bottoms, S.F., Rosen, M.G. and Dokol, R.J. (1980) The increase in the cesarean birth rate. *New England Journal of Medicine*, **302**: 559–562

[20] Grant, A., O'Brien, N., MacDonald, D., Joy, M.T., and Hennessey, E. (1989) Cerebral palsy among children born during the Dublin randomised trial of intrapartum monitoring. *Lancet*, **2**: 1233–1236.

Further reading

O'Driscoll, K. (1966) Rupture of the uterus. *Proceedings of the Royal Society of Medicine*, **59**: 65.

O'Driscoll, K., Foley, M., MacDonald, D. and Stronge, J. (1988) Cesarean section and perinatal outcome: Response from the House of Horne. *American Journal of Obstetrics and Gynaecology*, **158**: 499–452.

Turner, M.J., Rasmussen, M.J., Boylan, P.C., MacDonald, D. and Stronge, J. M. (1990) The influence of birth weight on labor in nulliparas. *Obstetrics and Gynecology*, **76**: 159–162.

Index